HEALTHY LIFESTYLE

Top Ten Preventable Causes of Premature Death with Real Stories of Change

Mohammad R. Torabi, Ph.D.
Kathy L. Finley, MS
Courtney O. Olcott, MS, MPH

authorHOUSE®

AuthorHouse™
1663 Liberty Drive
Bloomington, IN 47403
www.authorhouse.com
Phone: 1-800-839-8640

Published by AuthorHouse 4/29/2013

ISBN: 978-1-4817-1617-8 (sc)
ISBN: 978-1-4817-1616-1 (hc)
ISBN: 978-1-4817-1615-4 (e)

Library of Congress Control Number: 2013902818

TABLE OF CONTENTS

PREFACE

The leading causes of death of modern times in our industrialized society are heart disease, cancer, lung disease, stroke, diabetes, and HIV/AIDS. However, the actual causes of premature death, suffering, and morbidity are lifestyle related which include tobacco use, physical inactivity, poor nutrition, stress, and other lifestyle related factors. These factors are related to individual behaviors and decisions that cannot be necessarily dealt with by the medical community. These are public health issues which, to a great extent, are preventable. In contrast, about a century ago the leading causes of death were infectious diseases such as tuberculosis, influenza, etc. Consequently, the nature of the killers of modern time is different than the leading causes of death a hundred years ago. The strategy to deal with these lifestyle related health problems have to do with public health education, enactment, and enforcement of public health policies and access to preventive health care.

This book, in a non-technical and user friendly way, deals with eleven most preventable causes of premature death, disability, and morbidity. It also includes interviews with real individuals who have successfully dealt with lifestyle related factors like stress, nutrition, physical activity, tobacco, and other drug use, among others. This book is mainly designed for anyone with no or little background in health. Additionally, this introductory book includes applications and resources for gaining additional information so individuals can be empowered to make intelligent decisions with regard to adopting a healthy lifestyle.

Often we have heard that people think a healthy lifestyle is boring. The reality is when we, for example, include physical activity as a part of our daily routine, our immunity system will be enhanced, our work productivity will be improved, our outlook on life will be much more positive, and physically, intellectually, and emotionally we will feel much better as compared to adopting a sedentary lifestyle. Another example, tobacco is public health enemy number one which has no benefit whatsoever but has devastating health consequences not only on our physical health, but also on our emotional and mental health. Even tobacco will affect our gift of tasting food.

With regard to a healthy diet, one does not have to avoid the foods they like, but should have a balanced, adequate diet, rich in fruits and vegetables. Another example is stress which is obviously a major risk factor for the leading causes of death and it totally can be managed through education, skills, and intelligent decision-making.

These are examples of factors that have been covered in this book. Consequently, with adoption of a healthy lifestyle, one can expect higher life expectancy with quality vs. shorter life expectancy with illness and premature death. The authors sincerely believe that this book has a lot to offer to every member of our society.

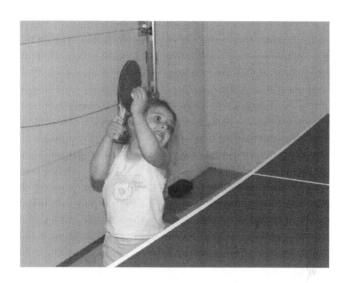

It is never too early or too late for adopting an active healthy lifestyle.

Mohammad R. Torabi, Ph.D.

STRESS

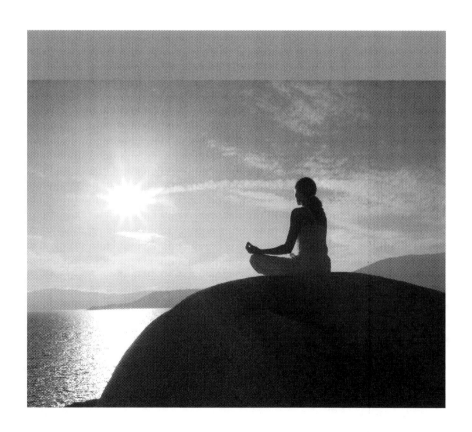

Stress is the "mental and physical response of our bodies to the changes and challenges" in life (Donatelle, 2010, p. 57). Stress can be chronic or acute. Stress is also categorized into good stress, also known as eustress, and bad stress, or distress (Donatelle, 2010). Stress can motivate people and help them meet goals. It can also overload people, causing physical, mental or behavioral problems, keeping them from accomplishing tasks. Each person reacts differently to stress. When individuals optimize stress, they are able to function in a balanced way. When individuals reach the point where stress no longer helps them meet goals, negative effects to their health may occur, including depression, anxiety, heart attack, stroke, hypertension, disturbance of immune system functioning, skin problems, gastrointestinal upset, and insomnia (American Institute of Stress, n.d.a). Costs associated with stress in the workplace include absenteeism, productivity loss, turnover, and healthcare. Approximately $300 billion annually is lost due to stress in the American workplace (Walach et al., 2007).

Sociocultural Influences

The concept of stress has evolved from scientists and social scientists weighing in on what stress is and what effects it has. Stress has been studied as an influence to a person's health since the 17th century (Cooper & Dewe, 2004). Robert Hooke, known as the Father of Modern Science in England during the 17th century, suggested stress in humans was similar to the concept of load in engineering. Hooke suggested the law of elasticity was similar to stress on the human body. In the law of elasticity, if a machine experiences a load, the machine will either be strong enough to sustain the load or succumb to the load and collapse or break down (Cooper & Dewe, 2004). Human body functioning was being likened to a machine's with the nervous system acting as the energy for the body; therefore, human bodies would also be susceptible to the effects of forces being placed upon them and break down or give way to wear and tear (Doublet, 2000).

Since 2006, the American Psychological Association (APA) has conducted an annual nationwide study on stress and its effects on Americans. The studies have uncovered the leading causes of stress, the stress-management behaviors being practiced, and the impact stress has. According to the 2007 study, one third of those studied reported that they experienced extreme stress. Nearly half of those studied reported that stress had a negative impact on their personal and professional lives while 77% reported having had physical symptoms from stress and 73% reported psychological symptoms from stress. The physical symptoms indicated in the study included: fatigue (51%), headache (44%), upset stomach (34%), muscle tension (30%), change in appetite (23%), teeth grinding (17%), change in sex drive (15%), and feeling dizzy (13%). The indicated psychological symptoms of their stress (APA, 2007) included: experiencing irritability or anger (50%), feeling nervous (45%), lack of energy (45%), and feeling as though one could cry (35%). Symptoms of stress reported by the 2010 survey included all of the physical symptoms from the 2007 survey as well as insomnia, sadness or depression, tightness in the chest, stomach upset, and change in appetite (APA, 2010). The study also found that individuals who reported higher levels of stress were more likely to be overweight or obese.

In 2010 (APA, 2010), nearly 40% of the study participants reported their stress had increased during the last five years. Money, work, and the economy were the most common sources of stress in the 2010 report. This study found that, in addition to serious economic struggles, Americans were overstressed due to trying to live a balanced lifestyle of healthy behaviors, work, and relationships.

Stages of Stress

Hans Selye, "The Father of Stress," was an internationally renowned physician who further investigated the concept of stress on the human body and how it related to physical illness (American Institute of Stress, n.d.b). In 1936, Selye illustrated the concept of stress with a model called the General Adaptation Syndrome (GAS). When individuals encounter a stressor, a physiological response sets into motion enabling them to deal with the stressor as they see fit. GAS describes this response using three phases: Alarm, Resistance, and Exhaustion (Selye, 1974, pp. 28-29). The Alarm Phase is described as the "fight or flight" response setting into action. This response is a series of chemical reactions causing the heart, blood pressure, and breathing rates to increase, allowing for a supply of energy to be available to muscles in order to fight or flee a danger (Donatelle, 2010). For example, when facing a mental stressor during the Alarm Phase, the stress-response system initiates the release of hormones that direct energy to the brain, so one can mentally address the stressful event; when facing a physical stressor, the stress-response system starts the release of hormones that supply muscles with the necessary oxygen and nutrients to fight that stressor (Donatelle, 2010).

In the Resistance Phase of GAS, the organs needed to fight or flee the stressor are still being utilized but to a lesser degree. During this phase, the body is attempting to return to a state of balance unless the threat of a stressor still exists. If the body cannot return to a state of balance, stress hormones continue to flow, leaving the body in a state of overarousal, eventually leading to the Exhaustion Phase (Donatelle, 2010). The Exhaustion Phase leads to wear and tear on the body because no relief from the stress response has occurred to allow the body to recover (McEwen, 2003). Individuals who experience chronic stress without allowing their body to return to a balanced state are at risk of developing stress-related health conditions.

Health Implications of Chronic Stress

Chronic, unpredictable or uncontrollable stress is more detrimental to a person's health than acute stress due to the continuous state of arousal of the body's stress response system (MedicineNet, 2011). Cardiovascular disease (CVD) is a serious health condition that can be brought on by or worsened by chronic stress (Donatelle, 2010). During GAS, the heart rate and blood pressure increase, and chronic high blood pressure causes hardening of the arteries, or atherosclerosis. It leads to damaged blood vessels and an increased risk for heart attack and stroke (Cohen, Janicki-Deverts, & Miller, 2007). All people, young and old, who experience chronic stress, are at risk for these effects.

In addition to risk for CVD, immune system functioning is suppressed during chronic stress. In the Exhaustion Phase, the body's immune response is compromised leaving the person more at risk of contracting illness or disease. The body's white blood cell count is lowered leaving the body less able to fight infection (Dugdale, 2009). A study examining data compiled over the last 30 years on stress management and immune system functioning illustrated how the body's immune system is negatively affected by acute or chronic stressors (Segerstrom & Miller, 2004).

Many other health issues can be attributed to chronic stress. Individuals may discover that pre-existing gastrointestinal issues or asthmatic conditions are worsened by it (Donatelle, 2010). Depression and anxiety can also result from it. Both are associated with stressful life situations like divorce, marital conflict, economic difficulties, and environmental factors (Katerndahl & Parchman, 2002). Stress can also play a role in causing headaches such as migraines and tension headaches (Insel & Roth, 2011).

Stress-Management Techniques

In order to prevent or reduce the negative effects on the body from stress, individuals can learn to better manage it. Stress-management techniques have been shown to reduce these effects (Insel & Roth, 2011). Studies show that other positive results from stress-management techniques include increased empathy and greater use of positive coping skills (Shapiro, Shapiro, & Schwarts, 2000). In addition, the techniques have been shown to improve blood sugar levels in type-2 diabetics and assist with the emotional and physical side effects of chemotherapy among cancer patients (Bennet & Carroll, 1990; Surwit et al., 2002).

Stress-management techniques apply different practices to calm the mind and body during stressful situations. A key to stress management is choosing healthy forms of it and avoiding dealing with stress in ways that increase risk factors for chronic diseases. When dealing with stress, individuals should avoid unhealthy behaviors, such as emotional eating or overeating, verbally or physically lashing out at others, and using tobacco, drugs, or alcohol. Instead, they should try out new stress-management techniques to determine which best fits their personal situation because a technique, such as meditation, may be successful for some but not for others (American Institute of Stress, n.d.a). Stress management can range in style from simple breathing techniques to listening to music or watching a funny movie or show (Donatelle, 2010).

Stress-management techniques recommended by medical professionals include daily exercise; a diet of fruit, vegetables, and whole grains; moderate alcohol use; no tobacco use; social support; yoga; meditation; and medications for chronic medical conditions (Cohen et al., 2007). Studies have shown that exercise increases white blood cell count, which assists immune systems in functioning well (Segerstrom & Miller, 2004). In addition, exercise burns off the by-products of the stress response system, so they will not lead to increased risk factors for disease or illness (Donatelle, 2010). Practicing daily stress management via exercise decreases risk factors associated with poor weight management, like diabetes,

CVD, or stroke; allows one to sleep better at night; and combats depression (Insel & Roth, 2011). Recent studies have shown that both stress management and exercise improve risk factors for CVD by increasing blood flow to the heart and decreasing blood pressure (Blumenthal et al., 2005).

Social support via friends, teachers, clergy, or family can also assist one through stressful life situations, minimizing the negative consequences of chronic stress (Bovier, Chamot, & Perneger, 2004). Relaxation techniques like yoga, Qigong, tai chi, deep breathing, meditation, progressive muscular relaxation, and massage therapy are also forms of stress management. Relaxation techniques work by slowing breathing and calming the body and mind. Other popular forms of stress management include journaling, participating in a hobby, drawing, playing an instrument, listening to music, humor, visualization, quiet time, and stretching.

For a personal point of view on coping with stress, we interviewed Jessica, a 29-year-old woman. For Jessica, stress is an everyday occurrence and comes in every incarnation, but her financial issues seem to be at the root of most of her stress. Stress causes Jessica to lose sleep, which is the biggest challenge she has associated with it because losing sleep creates more stress for her.

If the cause of stress is controllable, Jessica will try to change it; if the cause is inevitable, she learns to deal with it. That is how she successfully copes. But if she is not successful, Jessica can physically feel it in her neck and shoulders. The pain does not exist when she is calm and at ease. Music and exercise help place her in that state and deal with stress. Jessica also finds solace in a funny or relaxing television show. She realizes that none of those activities make the stressors disappear, but those momentary distractions may allow her to have a different perspective on them and possibly realize that there was nothing to be stressed about. Jessica notes that, if it is really bad, she can count on comfort food as a stress reliever.

For her personal perspective on stress management, we interviewed Lisa, a 25-year-old woman. As a student, Lisa is tense about writing papers, giving presentations, and studying. Recently, she had been very stressed during final exams. She was not able to sleep very much during that time and suffered from headaches, high blood pressure, and stomach problems. Lisa thought it was a living hell and she could not relax.

When Lisa is stressed, she angers easily and is mean to others even though she may care a lot about them. She also feels frustrated, pessimistic, and self-centered during times of high stress. Though she knows she is not the only one that feels this way, she feels lonely and will break down and cry. Lisa believes she has succeeded in coping with stress when she has received a good grade under pressure. She also feels good when she is able to finish projects without becoming sick. If she misses a regular workout in her exercise routine, she knows something is wrong. She also knows things have gone awry if she gets into an accident, hurts herself, or loses control. Unnecessary shopping is another indication of her not coping with stress effectively.

Lisa recommends healthy eating, sleeping at least seven hours per day, and exercising as effective behaviors to help cope with stress. Regular exercise also benefits her sleep schedule, which she tries to maintain. Eating healthy foods like salad and fruits make her feel more controlled and good. High fat and high sugar foods, which she wants when she is under stress, make her feel awful. Lisa combats the potential for unhealthy eating by preparing her lunch the night before, having a low-calorie snack bar handy, eating more fruits than sweets while studying or writing a paper, and choosing sugar-free candy and gum if she wants to eat when not hungry. Because Lisa gets upset when she is stressed, she tries to think about things that she has, things for which she is grateful, and that helps alleviate her stress level as well.

Conclusion

The release of stress hormones, such as cortisol, with no return to homeostasis can increase susceptibility to health problems such as CVD, immune system vulnerability, sleep disturbances, anxiety or depression, gastrointestinal conditions, headaches, and worsened asthma symptoms (Insel & Roth, 2011). Learning and utilizing stress-management techniques will benefit an individual's health. These techniques work to decrease stress symptoms by increasing blood flow to organs, relieving tension and chronic pain, improving concentration, reducing anger and frustration, and by lowering the heart rate, breathing rate, and blood pressure. Stress management allows people to live a healthier lifestyle both physically and emotionally.

Recommendations

Stress is a fact of life. Stress-management techniques allow people to handle it in a more positive way while decreasing risk factors for chronic disease or illness. A healthy balance of stress and stress management in life needs to be created in order to function well and avoid chronic stress-induced health conditions. Individuals should determine what is causing stress in their lives and manage these stressors by living a healthy lifestyle that includes regular exercise and sleep, a healthful diet, and relaxation techniques. Other steps to better manage stress include avoiding alcohol and tobacco, fostering healthy and supportive relationships, setting and keeping priorities, and maintaining a positive outlook (U.S. Department of Health and Human Services, 2009).

Evaluating the stressors in a person's life and dealing with them in constructive ways is an important strategy in decreasing health risk factors and managing stress. The following plan may assist individuals with that strategy:

1. Identify the stressor.

What is causing the distress? Time management issues, relationship problems, job stress, lack of physical exercise, or lack of quiet time are often at the base of stressful situations. Assess the stressors in your life and determine which unhealthy ways of coping need to be addressed.

2. Evaluate the stressor.

Is there too much emphasis on an event or situation? Is the stressor going to affect your future? Will the situation or stressor be important in one year, five years, or longer? Does the stressor need to be addressed immediately or can it wait?

3. Create a plan of action.

What can you do to manage the stressor(s)? You can attempt stress-management techniques to balance the effects of the stress response system. Is the stressor something that can be avoided? Can the stressor be dealt with straight on? Should the stressor be embraced?

4. Carry out the plan.

No matter what the stress-management plan is, be sure to carry it out to satisfaction. Begin the exercise program or meditation practice and stay with it. If you get off course, then you should get back to practicing the stress-management technique(s).

The following recommendations for an individual coping with stress are from the CDC (2009):

- **Stay in touch with family.** Stay around people who are caring and positive.
- **Stay active.** Go for a walk or run.
- **Get involved.** Get involved in activities to support your community.
- **Avoid drugs and alcohol.** Drugs and alcohol may seem to help with the stress temporarily; in the long run they create additional problems that compound the stress you are already feeling.
- **Find support.** Ask for help from a parent, friend, counselor, doctor, or pastor. Talk with them about the stress you feel and problems you face.
- **Take care of yourself.** Get plenty of rest and exercise and eat properly.
- **Take a time-out.** If you feel stressed, give yourself a break.

Allow some down time, even if it is only a 30-second time-out.

Selected Resources

The American Institute of Stress
124 Park Avenue
Yonkers, NY 10703
914-963-1200
Stress125@optline.net
www.stress.org/

American Psychological Association
750 First Street, NE
Washington, DC 20002
800-374-2721
www.apa.org/

Mayo Clinic
www.mayoclinic.com/health/stress-management/MY00435

National Institutes of Health
200 Independence Avenue
Washington, DC 20201
877-696-6775
www.nlm.nih.gov/medlineplus/stress.html

Substance Abuse and Mental Health Services Administration
1 Choke Cherry Road
Rockville, MD 20857
877-SAMHSA-7

References

American Institute of Stress. (n.d.a). Effects of stress. Retrieved February 28, 2011, from http://www.stress.org/topic-effects.htm

American Institute of Stress (n.d.b). Reminiscences of Hans Selye, and the birth of "stress." Retrieved March 26, 2011, from http://www.stress.org/hans.htm

American Psychological Association. (2007). Stress: A major problem in the U.S., warns APA. Retrieved March 2, 2011, from http://www.apa.org/news/press/releases/2007/10/stress.aspx

American Psychological Association. (2010). *Stress in America findings 2010.* Retrieved March 26, 2011, from http://www.apa.org/news/press/releases/stress/national-report.pdf

Bennet, P., & Carroll, D. (1990, February). Stress management approaches to the prevention of cardiovascular disease. *British Journal of Clinical Psychology*, 1-12.

Blumenthal, J. A., Sherwood, A. Babyak, M. A., Watkins, L. L., Waugh, R. Georgiades, A., . . . Hinderliter, A. (2005). Effects of exercise and stress management training on markers of cardiovascular risk in patients with ischemic heart disease. *Journal of the American Medical Association, 293*, 1626-1634.

Bovier, P. A., Chamot, E., & Perneger, T. V. (2004). Perceived stress, internal resources, and social support as determinants of mental health. *Quality of Life Research, 13*(1), 161-170.

Centers for Disease Control and Prevention. (2009). Coping with

stress. Retrieved on May 6, 2011, from http://www.cdc.gov/
Features/HandlingStress/

Cohen, S., Janicki-Deverts, D., & Miller, G. E. (2007). Psychological
stress and disease. *Journal of the American Medical Association,
298*(14), 1685-1687.

Cooper, C. L., & Dewe, P. (2004). *Stress: A brief history*. Oxford,
England: Blackwell.

Donatelle, R. J. (2010). *Health: The basics, Green edition*. San
Francisco, CA: Pearson Education.

Doublet, S. (2000). *The stress myth*. Freemans Reach NSW, Australia:
Ipsilon Publishing.

Dugdale, D. C. (2009). WBC count. Retrieved March 2, 2011, from
http://www.nlm.nih.gov /medlineplus/ency/article/003643.
htm

Insel, P. M., & Roth, W. T. (2011). *Connect core concepts in health*.
New York, NY: McGraw-Hill.

Katerndahl, D. A., & Parchman, M. (2002). The ability of the
stress process model to explain mental health outcomes.
Comprehensive Psychiatry, 43, 351-360.

McEwen, B. S. (2003). Mood disorders and allostatic load. *Biological
Psychiatry, 54*, 200-207.

MedicineNet. (2011). Stress. Retrieved March 26, 2011, from http://
www.medicinenet.com /stress/page8.htm

Segerstrom, S. C., & Miller, G. E. (2004). Psychological stress and
the human immune system: A meta-analytic study of 30 years
of inquiry. *Psychological Bulletin, 130*(4), 601-630.

Selye, H. (1974). *Stress without distress*. New York, NY: Lippincott.

Shapiro, S. L., Shapiro, D. E., & Schwarts, G. E. (2000). Stress management in medical education: A review of the literature. *Academic Medicine, 75*(7), 748-759.

Surwit, R. S., van Tilburg, M. A., Zucker, N., McCaskill, C. C., Priti, P., Feinglos, M. N., . . . Lane, J. D. (2002). Stress management improves long-term glycemic control in type 2 diabetes. *Diabetes Care, 25*(1), 30-34.

U.S. Department of Health and Human Services, Substance Abuse and Mental Health Services Administration. (2009). *Tips in a time of economic crisis: Managing your stress.* Retrieved March 31, 2011, from http://www.samhsa.gov/dtac/dbhis/dbhis_stress/pdf/SAMHSA_TipSheet_Manage%20Stress.pdf

Walach, H., Nord, E., Zier, C., Dietz-Waschkowski, B., Kersig, S., & Schupbach, H. (2007). Mindfulness based stress reduction as a method for personnel development: A pilot evaluation. *International Journal of Stress Management, 14*(2), 188-198.

NUTRITION

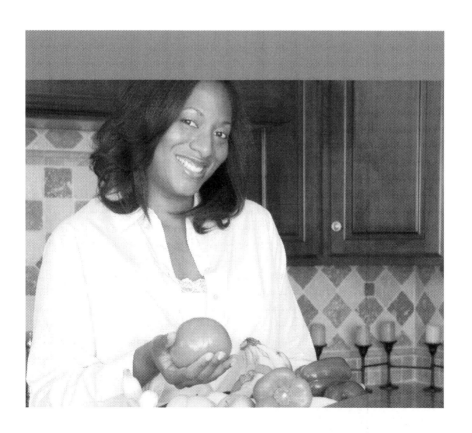

Nutrition is an integral part of human health. Proper nutrition provides energy for activities and learning. Eating healthful foods can assist with immune functioning and decrease the risk of chronic disease, such as heart disease, some types of cancer, osteoporosis, and diabetes (U.S. Department of Health and Human Services [HHS] & U.S. Department of Agriculture [USDA], 2010). Adequate nutritional or dietary intake can also aid weight management. As weight increases, even with moderate excess weight (10-20 lbs), so does the risk for premature death (HHS, 2001). In 2001, the Surgeon General's *Call to Action* stressed that obesity and overweight were at epidemic levels in the United States and asked for individuals to make more healthful decisions in their dietary intake and physical activity (HHS, 2001).

Sociocultural Influences

In 1969, the White House held its first event highlighting the importance of lifetime nutrition, the primary focus being on securing food for those suffering without it. This first meeting resulted in the expansion of the food stamp program and the creation of other programs such as the Special Supplemental Nutrition Program for Women, Infants, and Children (WIC), the school lunch program, and food labeling ("National Nutrition Summit," n.d.). In 1971, the first survey of Americans regarding nutritional intake, titled the National Health and Nutrition Surveys, was done. The surveys are still conducted on a yearly basis and information from them is used to study risk factors for disease and disease prevalence in the

US (CDC, 2009). The U.S. Dietary Guidelines, the first dietary recommendations for individuals 2 years and older, was established in 1980. These food choice recommendations are based on health promotion and disease prevention. In 1990, the U.S. Food and Drug Administration (FDA) was given the authority to control food labeling and the consistency of labeling terms.

In 2000, the meeting on nutrition was called the National Nutrition Summit and its focus was on nutrition in relation to the epidemic of overweight and obese Americans. Overweight or obesity are terms used to define weight that is more than normal and considered unhealthy based on an individual's height. The definitions for overweight and obesity are based on a scale called the body mass index (BMI). BMI is the relationship of an individual's weight to his or her height. Overweight is having a BMI of 25-29.9; obese is having a BMI of 30 or greater (CDC, 2010b). BMI can be used to determine a person's risk factor(s) for chronic disease (HHS, n.d.). Between 1976 and 1980, 46% of adult Americans were overweight or obese, and from 1988 to 1994, over 56% of them were overweight or obese. In addition, the increase in overweight children ages 6-18 was worrisome in regards to their lifelong health ("National Nutrition Summit," n.d.). Statistics from the 2007-2008 National Health and Nutrition Examination Survey show that approximately 34% of adults 20 and older were considered obese and 34% were considered overweight. In 2007-2008, obese adolescents were 18% of the population aged 12-19 years, while 20% of children 6-11 years of age were considered obese and 10% of youth 2-5 years of age were obese (CDC, 2010a). Currently, the U.S. Surgeon General's *Vision for a Healthy and Fit Nation* sets forth a plan to get Americans to engage in physical activity on a daily basis, manage stress, and choose nutritious foods (HHS & USDA, 2010).

The perception of food has slowly changed. Food is a form of entertainment now as well as energy intake. In the US today, there are more restaurants and families eating out than before 1977. Between 1977 and 1991, eating establishments increased by 75%

(CDC, 2006). The daily calories eaten at establishments away from home have increased since the 1970s (CDC, 2006; Stewart, Blisard, & Jolliffe, 2006). Frequency of eating out is associated with an increase in calorie and fat intake and BMI (CDC, 2006). Individuals who eat out more often are at an increased risk of weight gain and being overweight or obese, especially when a person eats one or more meals at fast food establishments weekly (HHS & USDA, 2010). Further, individuals who live in communities with a large number of fast food restaurants tend to have a higher BMI than those living in communities with less fast food restaurants.

Other changes in the American environment have also played a role in the increase in obese and overweight Americans. Between 1970 and the present, the food supply has increased in all food categories, causing an increase in the number of calories for each person by 600 calories. An increase in caloric intake can lead to increased weight, contributing to larger numbers of overweight and obese people in the US (USDA, 2010). Portion sizes have also increased, and research indicates the larger the portion size a person is served, the more the person will eat. Large portion sizes are linked to increased body weight; smaller portion sizes are linked to a decrease in body weight (HHS & USDA, 2010).

In addressing the issue of obese and overweight people in America, physical activity and nutritional intake have become the two focal points for the U.S. Department of Health and Human Services (HHS) and the U.S. Department of Agriculture (USDA). Nutritional intake influences weight, risk for chronic disease, and the promotion of overall health (HHS & USDA, 2010). A special emphasis has been placed on healthy eating for young children ages 2 years and older. Young children in the United States are eating foods that are low in nutrient density and high in calories. Unhealthy childhood eating habits lead to increased risk factors for chronic disease in children that are normally seen in adults, and food habits often carry into adulthood. Healthy eating habits along with an increase in physical activity are crucial to combat the epidemic of obesity and overweight people in the United States (HHS & USDA, 2010).

Caloric Intake

Nutritional intake provides the body with the calories, or energy, needed for organs to function. Calories come from carbohydrates, protein, or fat. Each body requires a baseline amount of calories in order to support basic life functions. Caloric needs beyond the baseline amount are based on gender, body composition (height and weight), and caloric output (physical activity). Caloric need estimates are 1,600-2,400 calories per day for adult women and 2,000-3,000 calories per day for adult men. Child and adolescent caloric need estimates are 1,400-3,200 calories per day with males generally requiring a higher caloric intake (HHS & USDA, 2010). The goal regarding nutritional intake is to find a caloric balance between what a person needs and what a person burns on a regular basis. People who balance calories taken in with calories burned will hold a consistent weight (CDC, 2006). Currently in America, two thirds of adults are overweight or obese and one in every three children are obese or overweight (Flegal, Carroll, Ogden, & Curtin, 2010; Ogden, Carroll, Curtin, Lamb, & Flegal, 2010). Clearly a balance between calories taken in and calories burned does not exist in many Americans' lives. Reasons for the increase in overweight or obese Americans include activity level and the types of food and amount they eat on a regular basis, including increased portion sizes (CDC, 2006; HHS & USDA, 2010).

Recommended Dietary Intake

According to the National Cancer Institute (n.d.b), some of the top sources of caloric intake in the US include grains-based desserts, pizza, soda, alcohol, pasta and pasta dishes, dairy desserts, tortillas or tacos, burgers, potato/corn/other chips, candy, whole milk, fried white potatoes, fruit drinks, sausage/hot dogs/bacon/ribs, beef or beef-mixed dishes, pancakes or waffles, and crackers. Foods such as these are high in calories and low in nutrients, increasing the risk for overweight or obese consumers and thereby increasing their risk for chronic disease.

The HHS and the USDA create new dietary guidelines for Americans every five years. The dietary guidelines include recommendations for health promotion, disease reduction, and weight management. Consuming a varied and balanced diet high in whole grains, fruit and vegetables, lean proteins, low-fat dairy products, and healthy fats will aid weight management while working to prevent chronic diseases like cardiovascular disease (CVD), high blood pressure, diabetes, osteoporosis, and some types of cancer (HHS & USDA, 2010).

The HHS and USDA daily recommended sources of calories are carefully laid out in the Choose My Plate format (USDA, n.d). Choose My Plate is a plate-shaped icon that guides people in making food choices that are nutrient filled and health promoting when eaten in the appropriate amounts. Choose My Plate consists of five sections in varying sizes representing the recommended amounts of five different food groups: grains, proteins, fruits, vegetables, and dairy. Choose My Plate also makes personalized suggestions for daily recommended servings from each of the food groups based on individual needs.

Choose My Plate illustrates that the majority of an individual's caloric needs should be satisfied by the grains group. Examples of grains include any food made from wheat, rice, oats, or barley, such as cereal, bread, oatmeal, pasta, or tortillas. For health promotion, evidence supports having half the grains come from whole grain products (HHS & USDA, 2010). Whole grains contain fiber and fiber helps reduce blood cholesterol levels, which may reduce the risk of CVD. In addition, adults who eat more whole grains have a lower body weight compared to adults who eat a lower number of whole grains (American Heart Association, 2011).

Whole grains can be found in commonly found products such as oatmeal, popcorn, barley, and brown rice. Many products containing whole grains exist, but, sometimes, shopping for whole grains can be difficult because product labeling can be misleading. Products named *wheat bread* or *wheat buns* can contain enriched flour instead of whole grains. To check whether a product is truly whole wheat or whole grain, a person can search the ingredient label on the package for any of the following words: *whole grain, whole wheat, whole rye, whole grain cornmeal,* and *whole wheat pasta.* If the word *enriched* is on the ingredient label, then the product is not a whole grain and therefore will not provide the benefits of whole grains. Most enriched products have had important vitamins and minerals removed in the milling process, which creates a finer texture and a longer shelf life but does not promote health. While some vitamins are added back into the product later, fiber is left out (USDA, n.d.).

Fruits and vegetables are two separate sections of Choose My Plate. Fruits and vegetables are low in calories and high in nutrients, promoting a healthy weight. In addition, fruit and vegetable intake has been associated with a lower risk for CVD, heart attack, stroke, type 2 diabetes, and some types of cancer (HHS & USDA, 2010). In America, intake from these two food groups is lower than recommended, leaving people with a lack of vital vitamins and minerals, such as folate, magnesium, potassium, dietary fiber, and vitamins A, K, and C. Potassium-filled fruits, like prunes, bananas, and cantaloupe, help to maintain healthy blood pressure. Dietary fiber leaves the consumer feeling fuller and eating fewer calories while working to reduce cholesterol levels and lower heart disease risk (USDA, n.d.). Fruits and vegetables with vitamin A aid in the health of eyes and skin while protecting against infection. Fruits and vegetables high in vitamin C assist body tissues with growth and repair, helping to heal wounds and keep gums healthy. Vitamin E comes from food sources such as broccoli, almonds, sunflower seeds or oil, spinach, vegetable oil, kiwi, mangoes, tomatoes, peanuts, and soybean oil (National Institutes of Health, 2010). Vitamin E is an antioxidant and important in protecting vitamin A and fatty acids from cell oxidation. Cell oxidation is the process associated with the development of cancer (National Cancer Institute, 2010a), so warding off cell oxidation is crucial in preventing or slowing some types of cancer (Blott et al., 1993).

Some evidence does suggest that antioxidants from vegetables or fruits may have this effect on cancer (National Cancer Institute, n.d.a). In 1993, the first randomized study examining the influence of antioxidants on cancer was done in China, and it found that the incidence of gastric and overall cancer was lower in males and females who ingested regular amounts of antioxidants such as beta-carotene, selenium, and vitamin E (Blott et al., 1993). Antioxidants can be found in large quantities in fruits and vegetables and in lower amounts in meat, poultry, fish, grains, and nuts.

Evidence supports eating a wide variety of fruits and vegetables and focusing on different colors of them throughout a person's diet. Beverages containing 100% fruit or vegetable juice can count as a fruit or vegetable serving, but Choose My Plate recommends only one serving each of a person's recommended daily fruit and vegetable intake be ingested in this form as juice lacks fiber and is higher in calories than fruit or vegetables. Fruits and vegetables can be consumed whole, raw, mashed, pureed, frozen, dried, or cut up (USDA, n.d.). Mixing fruits or vegetables in other foods is a great way to increase consumption of both food groups. Fruit can be easily mixed into smoothies, oatmeal, yogurts, or cereals, and vegetables can be mashed or pureed into drinks, casseroles, or other recipes.

Dairy is another section of Choose My Plate. Dairy includes any product made from milk that maintains its calcium content. Examples of items made from milk that are excluded from the dairy group include butter, cream, and cream cheese. The dairy servings should consist of low- to non-fat products with little to no added sugar. Dairy products contain important nutrients like calcium, vitamin D, and potassium. Calcium is important for bone density and bone growth. Vitamin D helps to keep calcium and phosphorous levels constant in the body, helping to maintain bone density and strength (USDA, n.d.). Vitamin D is also important for healthy immune system functioning and nerve conduction for muscles. Vitamin D is currently being studied to determine if there is a connection between lack of vitamin D and diabetes, hypertension, autoimmune disorder, cancer, or multiple sclerosis (National Institutes of Health, 2011).

Protein sources make up the next section of Choose My Plate. Protein sources include meat, poultry, fish, dry beans or peas, eggs, nuts, and seeds. Lean protein sources are recommended, including nuts and seeds, which contain healthy oils and fats. Serving size recommendations differ based on individual needs, and it is recommended people eat a variety of protein sources. Cholesterol is found in animal sources of protein and Choose My Plate recommends limiting the amount of cholesterol in a person's diet as high cholesterol increases the risk for CVD (USDA, n.d.).

Protein sources contain many healthful vitamins and nutrients. Protein itself is vital to building muscle, bones, cartilage, skin, and blood. In addition, protein is needed for hormones, enzymes, and vitamins to function properly. Iron present in protein sources carries oxygen to body tissues, and magnesium is used for bone building and energy for muscle function. Protein sources also provide zinc, which aids in immune system functioning. The vitamins B and E found in protein sources assist with tissue repair, the release of energy, the functioning of the nervous system and red blood cell formation (USDA, n.d.).

Healthy fats or oils are also included as a section in Choose My Plate. This section is the smallest of Choose My Plate as intake of oils should be minimal compared to the other food groups listed. The consumption of unsaturated fats, like polyunsaturated or monounsaturated oils and fats, are vital to a health-promoting diet (HHS & USDA, 2010). Healthy oils or fats include the following: canola, corn, cottonseed, olive, safflower, soybean, and sunflower. Healthy oils containing unsaturated fats are good for a person's health because they improve cholesterol levels, decrease inflammation, and help with heart rhythms, all working to decrease risk of CVD (Harvard School of Public Health, n.d.). Solid fats are high in saturated fats. Both saturated and trans fats should be limited in a person's dietary intake. Diets high in saturated fats lead to poor cholesterol levels, increasing LDLs (bad cholesterol), and the risk for CVD (USDA, n.d.).

Consumers can identify trans fats in food products by reading the nutrition ingredient label and looking for the words *hydrogenated* or *partially-hydrogenated*. If either word appears on the ingredient label, then the food contains trans fats. Trans fats cause inflammation damage to the blood vessels, increase LDLs (bad cholesterol), lower HDLs (good cholesterol), and increase triglycerides, all of which increase the risk of CVD (Mayo Clinic staff, 2009).

Added Sugars and Sodium

Many health professionals are concerned about the added sugars and sodium within the American diet that increase risk factors for CVD and being overweight or obese. Added sugars and sodium account for 30% of the American diet and provide no nutrients or health promotion. Added sugars pose health concerns via extra calories in a person's diet. Added sugars, composing about 16% of the American diet, are those that are added into foods, not the naturally occurring sugars like the fructose found in fruits or lactose found in milk (HHS & USDA, 2010). Currently, most Americans ages 2 years and older consume 3,200 mg of sodium daily. Sodium intake for the average American should be limited to 2,300 mg daily. Increased sodium intake raises blood pressure, which is a risk factor for CVD, congestive heart failure, and kidney disease (HHS & USDA, 2010).

We interviewed David, a 37-year-old man, for his experience with nutrition. David doesn't feel like nutrition was a matter of great importance to his parents. Besides corn on the cob, he didn't eat fresh vegetables growing up. Instead, he ate and still enjoys foods like pizza and Mexican dishes. David had never thought about what he ate until college. Being married now and planning to have a family of his own has made him more conscious of the importance of eating well.

As David continues his studies, his full work schedule challenges his eating behavior. He doesn't often feel like he has the time to fix a good meal or find healthy alternatives. Food is almost treated like fuel because he needs to eat and go. Another obstacle to eating healthier is that the food he likes and grew up on is not very good for him. In the year before our interview, David discovered his sugar levels were at a near-diabetic state, necessitating a drastic diet change. He believes the change has been a success for the most part, but he concedes that he doesn't follow his diet every time he eats and that he still has late-night cravings for chocolate.

David feels he has succeeded in improving his nutrition because he is more conscious of his food choices, knowing that, if he eats unhealthily one night, he needs to eat better in the surrounding days. But David has not lost as much weight as he needs to, and he recognizes that his diet is ongoing, not just for two or three months. For those who would like to know more about nutrition, David suggests for them to speak openly with their doctors and be truthful about their choices. He also recommends setting attainable goals and rewarding oneself for weight loss by buying new clothes to fit the slimmer body.

For a personal point of view and experience with nutrition, we interviewed Brian, a 32-year-old man. Brian's interest in nutrition began about 15 years ago. He became a vegan, but after more than a year as one, the lifestyle made him feel unhealthy. He started learning more about nutrition then and tried high protein diets, which worked for him. Brian also stopped eating sugar for long stretches of time. Then, four or five years ago, he discovered a book on the blood type diet, a diet he had always been skeptical about. When he examined the diet further, it seemed to make sense to him. The blood type diet instructed him to eat red meat and he did so, feeling better afterward. For him, the most difficult part of nutrition is understanding what to believe. Brian believes the benefits of all food are readily available and that there is a wealth of theories on food. The blood type diet tied everything together for him.

Brian feels that he has found success in this aspect of his life because he has energy, is not overweight, and does not feel overly tired after meals. He suggests that people try a few fad diets first and see how they feel. Then, he recommends trying the blood type diet and following it faithfully for a couple of weeks. He thinks that anyone would notice a difference, but he also believes people eat the right foods for themselves instinctually. Brian promotes the blood type diet as great for people who have been desensitized to how they feel while eating. He feels that a positive outcome of the blood type diet is that, after being on it for some time, individuals may easily feel the difference when eating food that is not good for them like he does, and he believes that having that sensitivity of knowing themselves in that way is incredible.

Conclusion

Health-promoting dietary intake includes a balance of calories taken in with physical activity. It also includes variety in food intake that focuses on whole grains, fruits and vegetables, low- to non-fat dairy products, lean meats or protein sources with healthy oils, and an increase in mono and polyunsaturated fats while decreasing saturated fat intake and trans fats intake. In addition, intake of added sugars and sodium should be reduced to lower risk factors for CVD, overweight or obesity, diabetes, and other chronic health conditions. Caloric need differs from person to person based on gender, age, physical activity, and body composition; therefore, serving size from each food group also differs from person to person. People should know their approximate caloric needs in order to maintain a balance in calories ingested with physical activity.

Recommendations

Recommended daily allowances for each of the food groups in Choose My Plate are set by the USDA Center for Nutrition Policy and Promotion (CNPP). The CNPP is in charge of making nutrition recommendations to Americans based on scientific research. The

Choose My Plate website will individualize food group serving sizes based on a healthy person's gender, physical activity level, and age. General population Choose My Plate recommendations include food group servings for each of the following groups: children ages 2-3 and 4-8; girls 9-13 and 14-18; boys 9-13 and 14-18; women 19-30, 31-50, and 51+ years; and men 19-30, 31-50 and 51+ years (USDA, 2011). Servings are recommended in the form of either cups or ounces depending on the food group. Examples of an ounce of grain include 1 slice of bread, 1 cup of ready-to-eat cereal, and ½ cup of cooked rice, cooked pasta, or cooked cereal (USDA, n.d.). Examples of a serving size of protein include an ounce of meat, poultry, or fish, ¼ cup of cooked dry beans, 1 egg, 1 tablespoon of peanut butter, or a ½ ounce of nuts or seeds (USDA, n.d.).

The following are general serving guidelines from the USDA (n.d.) for individuals with no chronic medical conditions. Guidelines for the grains group include the recommendations that half of total grain intake should come from whole grains. Each serving size listed is the recommended amount for the age and gender specified per day.

Grains

Children	Women
2-3 years of age 3 ounces	19-30 years of age 6 ounces
4-8 years of age 4-5 ounces	31-50 years of age 6 ounces
	51+ years of age 5 ounces
Girls	
9-13 years of age 5 ounces	**Men**
14-18 years of age 6 ounces	19-30 years of age 8 ounces
	31-50 years of age 7 ounces
Boys	51+ years of age 6 ounces
9-13 years of age 6 ounces	
14-18 years of age 7 ounces	

Vegetables

Children	Women
2-3 years of age 1 cup	19-30 years of age 2 ½ cups
4-8 years of age 1 ½ cups	31-50 years of age 2 ½ cups
	51+ years of age 2 cups
Girls	
9-13 years of age 2 cups	**Men**
14-18 years of age 2 ½ cups	19-30 years of age 3 cups
	31-50 years of age 3 cups
Boys	51+ years of age 2 ½ cups
9-13 years of age 2 ½ cups	
14-18 years of age 3 cups	

Fruit

Children	Women
2-3 years of age 1 cup	19-30 years of age 2 cups
4-8 years of age 1 to 1 ½ cups	31-50 years of age 1 ½ cups
	51+ years of age 1 ½ cups
Girls	
9-13 years of age 1 ½ cups	**Men**
14-18 years of age 1 ½ cups	19-30 years of age 2 cups
	31-50 years of age 2 cups
Boys	51+ years of age 2 cups
9-13 years of age 1 ½ cups	
14-18 years of age 2 cups	

Dairy

Children	Women
2-3 years of age 2 cups	19-30 years of age 3 cups
4-8 years of age 2 cups	31-50 years of age 3 cups
	51+ years of age 3 cups
Girls	
9-13 years of age 3 cups	**Men**
14-18 years of age 3 cups	19-30 years of age 3 cups
	31-50 years of age 3 cups
Boys	51+ years of age 3 cups
9-13 years of age 3 cups	
14-18 years of age 3 cups	

Protein

Children	Women
2-3 years of age 2 ounces	19-30 years of age 5 ½ ounces
4-8 years of age 3-4 ounces	31-50 years of age 5 ounces
	51+ years of age 5 ounces
Girls	
9-13 years of age 5 ounces	**Men**
14-18 years of age 5 ounces	19-30 years of age 6 ½ ounces
	31-50 years of age 6 ounces
Boys	51+ years of age 5 ½ ounces
9-13 years of age 5 ounces	
14-18 years of age 6 ounces	

Selected Resources

Centers for Disease Control and Prevention
Division of Nutrition, Physical Education, and Obesity
1600 Clifton Road
Atlanta, GA 30333
800-CDC-INFO (800-232-4636)
www.cdc.gov/nccdphp/dnpao/

Harvard School of Public Health
677 Huntington Avenue
Boston, MA 02115
www.hsph.harvard.edu/nutritionsource/

Institute of Medicine of the National Academies
500 Fifth Street, NW
Washington, DC 20001
202-334-2352
www.iom.edu/Global/Topics/Food-Nutrition.aspx

National Institutes of Health
Division of Nutrition Research Coordination
6707 Democracy Boulevard
Room 624, MSC 5461
Bethesda, MD 20892-5450
301-594-8822
dnrc.nih.gov/

U.S. Department of Agriculture
Center for Nutrition Policy and Promotion
3101 Park Center Drive
10th Floor
Alexandria, VA 22302-1594
888-7-PYRAMID
www.ChooseMyPlate.gov/index.html

References

American Heart Association. (2011). Whole grains and fiber. Retrieved February 24, 2011, from http://www.heart.org/HEARTORG/ GettingHealthy/NutritionCenter/HealthyDietGoals/Whole-Grains-and-Fiber_UCM_303249_Article.jsp

Blot, W. J., Li, J. Y., Taylor, P. R., Guo, W., Dawsey, S., Wang, C. Q., . . . Li, B. (1993). Nutrition intervention trials in Linxian, China: Supplementation with specific vitamin/mineral combinations, cancer incidence, and disease-specific mortality in the general population. *Journal of the National Cancer Institute, 85*(18), 1483-1491.

Centers for Disease Control and Prevention. (2010a). FastStats: Obesity and overweight. Retrieved March 11, 2011, from http:// www.cdc.gov/nchs/fastats/overwt.htm

Centers for Disease Control and Prevention. (2010b). Overweight and obesity: Defining overweight and obesity. Retrieved May 3, 2011, from http://www.cdc.gov/obesity/defining.html

Centers for Disease Control and Prevention, Division of Nutrition and Physical Activity. (2006). *Research to practice series no. 2: Portion size.* Atlanta, GA: Author.

Centers for Disease Control and Prevention, National Center for Health Statistics. (2009). About the National Health and Nutrition Examination Survey. Retrieved March 11, 2011, from http://www.cdc.gov/nchs/nhanes/about_nhanes.htm

Flegal, K. M., Carroll, M. D., Ogden, C. L., & Curtin, L. R. (2010). Prevalence and trends in obesity among US adults, 1999-2008. *Journal of the American Medical Association, 303*(3), 235-241.

Harvard School of Public Health. (n.d.). The Nutrition Source - Fats and cholesterol: Out with the bad, in with the good. Retrieved February 27, 2011, from http://www.hsph.harvard.edu/nutritionsource/what-should-you-eat/fats-full-story/index.html

Mayo Clinic staff. (2009). High cholesterol. Retrieved February 27, 2011, from http://www.mayoclinic.com/health/trans-fat/CL00032/NSECTIONGROUP=2

National Cancer Institute. (n.d.a). Antioxidants and cancer prevention: Fact sheet. Retrieved March 22, 2011, from http://www.cancer.gov/cancertopics/factsheet/prevention/antioxidants#r1

National Cancer Institute. (n.d.b). Risk factor monitoring and methods - Cancer control and population sciences: Food sources. Retrieved from http://riskfactor.cancer.gov /diet/foodsources/

National Institutes of Health, Office of Dietary Supplements. (2010). Dietary supplement fact sheet: Vitamin E. Retrieved May 4, 2011, from http://ods.od.nih.gov/factsheets/VitaminE-QuickFacts/

National Institutes of Health, Office of Dietary Supplements. (2011). Dietary supplement fact sheet: Vitamin D. Retrieved May 4, 2011, from http://ods.od.nih.gov/factsheets /VitaminD-QuickFacts/

National Nutrition Summit 2000 - Background brief: Purpose of the National Nutrition Summit. (n.d.). Retrieved March 11, 2011, from http://www.nns.nih.gov/2000/background/background_brief/brief.htm

Ogden, C. L., Carroll, M. D., Curtin, L. R., Lamb, M. M., & Flegal, K. M. (2010). Prevalence of high body mass index in US children and adolescents, 2007-2008. *Journal of the American Medical Association, 303*(3), 242-249.

Stewart, H., Blisard, N., & Jolliffe, D. (2006). *Let's eat out: Americans weigh taste, convenience, and nutrition.* Retrieved March 11, 2011, from http://www.ers.usda.gov/publications/eib19/eib19.pdf.

U.S. Department of Agriculture. (n.d.). ChooseMyPlate.gov. Retrieved from http://www.choosemyplate.gov

U.S. Department of Agriculture. (2010). Food availability (per capita) data system. Retrieved August 12, 2010, from http://www.ers.usda.gov/Data/FoodConsumption/

U.S. Department of Agriculture, Center for Nutrition Policy and Promotion. (2011). Center for Nutrition Policy and Promotion: Improving the nutrition and well-being of Americans. Retrieved March 25, 2011, from http://www.cnpp.usda.gov/

U.S. Department of Health and Human Services, National Institutes of Health, National Heart, Lung, and Blood Institute. (n.d.). Calculate your body mass. Retrieved March 9, 2011, from http://www.nhlbisupport.com/bmi/

U.S. Department of Health and Human Services, Public Health Service, Office of the Surgeon General. (2001). *The Surgeon General's call to action to prevent and decrease overweight and obesity.* Washington, DC: Government Printing Office.

U.S. Department of Health and Human Services & U.S. Department of Agriculture. (2010). *Dietary guidelines for Americans, 2010* (7th ed.). Retrieved March 9, 2011, from http://www.health.gov/dietaryguidelines/

PHYSICAL ACTIVITY

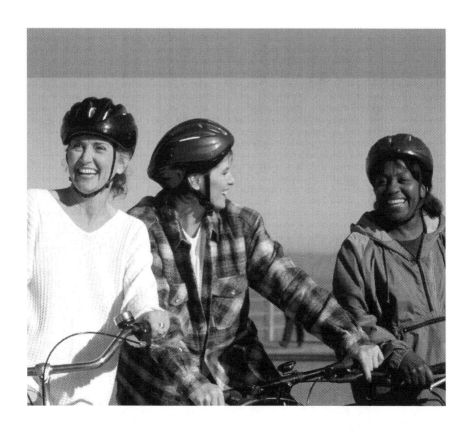

Physical activity is any action beyond normal body movement for daily functioning (U.S. Department of Health and Human Services [HHS], 2009). It includes actions such as walking, running, jumping, playing, gardening, swimming, and much more. A person's physical health and well-being can benefit from physical activity. Health promotion occurs when it is done in varying—moderate and/or vigorous—degrees of intensity. Physical activity should also include aerobic, muscle-strengthening, and bone-strengthening activities (HHS, 1996). A goal of physical activity is to improve one's level of physical fitness, which incorporates cardiovascular health, body composition, strength, and endurance (HHS, President's Council on Physical Fitness and Sports, 2000).

Everyone can benefit from regular physical activity, but currently, about one third of Americans do not participate in any regular physical activity (Centers for Disease Control and Prevention [CDC], 2008). Lack of physical activity is associated with chronic diseases, such as heart disease, some types of cancer, stroke, high blood pressure, type 2 diabetes, and obesity (CDC, 2003; HHS, 2008). In 2007, only 1 of the 50 states had an obesity rating of less than 20%, and as of 2009, no state had met the Healthy People 2010 objective of an obesity rating of less than 15% (CDC, 2010b). Because sedentary lifestyles lead to a higher risk of obesity and because more than 72 million U.S. adults are obese, physical activity is vital to U.S. public health (CDC, 2010b).

Sociocultural Influences

Physical activity has been a part of survival from the beginning of time for man (Dalleck & Kravitz, 2002). Hundreds of years ago, people hunted for their own food, prepared it, and made clothing and shelter for themselves. They did not have to think about physical activity because from dawn to dusk it was a fact of life. In the United States, physical activity has come and gone in popularity or necessity throughout the years. During the Colonial Period, life was difficult for settlers, requiring much physical activity in order to have food and shelter. Physical activity was encouraged by President Thomas Jefferson during the National Period in the US. After the Civil War, when industrialization boomed, the physical activity required to survive began to diminish. More people used machines in the place of hard labor, so physical activity lessened. Required physical education in the schools resulted from the fact that many Americans were found to be out of shape and unfit for the military during World War I (Dalleck & Kravitz, 2002).

The 1920s brought on a new mentality of relaxation and entertainment. Funding was nonexistent for physical education programming and the enthusiasm for physical activity diminished leading to more unfit Americans attempting to enter the military during World War II. Continued lack of physical activity in American culture was illuminated when fitness testing on U.S. children was conducted during the 1950s. Approximately 60% of U.S. children failed physical strength and flexibility testing forcing the U.S. government to create the President's Council on Youth Fitness and the President's Citizens-Advisory Committee on Fitness of American Youth. Several professional agencies focusing on the importance of physical activity were created during the 1950s, including the well-respected American College of Sports Medicine (ACSM) in 1954. In addition, during this time in history, Dr. Ken Cooper, "the Father of the Modern Fitness Movement," continued to promote and gain support for physical activity as a way to maintain health and prevent disease (Dalleck & Kravitz, 2002).

Today, Americans face new challenges in fitting physical activity into their daily lives. Many modern conveniences have allowed people to complete work by sitting in front of a computer or by standing still for many hours at a time. The health cost from this shift to less daily physical activity is chronic disease, decreased quality of life, expensive health management, and premature death. Lack of physical activity can be linked to 4 of the top 10 leading causes of death and disease in the United States: cardiovascular disease (CVD), some types of cancer, stroke, and diabetes (CDC, 2009a; Flegal, Carroll, Ogden, & Curtin, 2010). Obesity is a major contributing factor to each of them. The annual direct and indirect economic costs in Medicare and Medicaid from obesity-related diseases topped $78 billion in 1998 and $147 billion in 2006. Individuals who were overweight in 2006 had $1,429 more in health-related costs annually than those who were not overweight (CDC, 2009b; Finkelstein, Trogden, Cohen, & Dietz, 2009).

Biology and Physiology

A person suffering from obesity has a body mass index (BMI) of 30 or greater while an overweight person has a BMI over 25. BMI is calculated from a person's weight and height and is often used to illustrate a person's risk for developing obesity-related chronic disease (CDC, 2010a). The number of obese and overweight adults in the US has increased from 15% (1976-1980 survey) to 32% (2003-2004 survey). Obesity rates in 2007-2008 did not grow at the previous rate but were still high at 32.2% for adult men and 35.5% for adult women (Flegal et al., 2010).

Adults are not the only ones at risk of developing obesity-related chronic disease. Sedentary children have an increased risk of becoming overweight or obese, and those considered overweight or obese show greater incidents of high blood pressure, high blood cholesterol levels, and type 2 diabetes compared to those not overweight or obese (HHS, n.d.). The 2007-2008 National Health and Nutrition Examination Survey (NHANES) showed that an estimated 16.9% of U.S. children between 2-19 years of age were obese (as cited in Ogden, Carroll, Curtin, Lamb, & Flegal, 2010). Studies also concluded that a majority of children overweight or obese during their youth will be obese or overweight into their adulthood (Daniels et al., 2005).

Physical activity levels decrease as a child ages. Youth aged 6-7 years participate in approximately 46 minutes of physical activity per day whereas youth 10-16 years of age are physically active between 16-45 minutes per day with males being 20% more active than females (American Academy of Pediatrics, 2006). Reasons youth give for inactivity include inactive role models or parents, competing demands/pressures, unsafe environments, lack of recreation facilities, and inadequate access to physical education (American Academy of Pediatrics, 2006).

Physical activity has many health benefits. It reduces risk of CVD, stroke, type 2 diabetes, metabolic syndrome, and some types of cancers, and it manages weight, strengthens bones and muscles, improves mental health and mood, increases the chance for a longer life span, and decreases risk of falls among older adults (CDC, 2011; HHS, 2008). Health benefits for youth include improved aerobic fitness, mood, and self esteem; continued physical activity into adulthood; muscular strength; improved BMI, blood lipid profile, and blood pressure; a decrease in the degree of overweight in obese children; and improved fitness in obese and overweight children (CDC, 1997).

Physical activity benefits cardiovascular health by increasing the body's ability to handle and transport oxygen. The heart is made of muscle and regular physical activity improves the circulatory and muscle functions of the heart (Myers, 2003). Improvement in diabetes risk is seen with regular physical activity because it enhances the body's ability to use glucose (American Diabetes Association, n.d.). Regular physical activity helps to manage weight by using energy and creating or maintaining muscle, thereby burning calories and decreasing the risk of both cardiovascular disease and diabetes (Thompson, 2011). Physical activity boosts endorphins in the bloodstream that help to reduce anxiety and improve mood. It also helps to boost immune system functioning (Mayo Clinic staff, 2009a). Further, physical activity improves cholesterol profiles by increasing good cholesterol (high density lipoproteins) and decreasing bad cholesterol (low density lipoproteins). It also decreases resting blood pressure, improving risk factors for circulatory disease (Donatelle, 2010). Improvements in physical activity will also positively influence a person's mortality rate. One study indicates a 44% reduction in mortality among individuals who went from unfit to fit via regular physical activity over a five-year period (Warburton, Nicol, & Bredin, 2006).

Components of Physical Activity

Regular physical activity is necessary to a healthy lifestyle (HHS, Office of the Surgeon General, n.d.). It has many components to consider, so when people plan to increase their physical activity or begin an exercise program, they should always discuss it with a health-care provider and remember that the main point is to get moving through overload, progression, and specificity (HHS, 2008). Overload focuses on the amount and intensity of physical activity, requiring more physical stress than usual from the body. Progression requires the person to move to higher levels of physical stress as the body adapts to new levels of cardiorespiratory fitness. Specificity indicates that benefits from the physical activity will be specific to the organs being worked (HHS, 2008).

The three types of activity to focus on for health benefits are aerobic, muscle strengthening, and bone strengthening. Aerobic physical activity includes actions, like running, biking, or swimming, that require the body's large muscles to be active for a sustained amount of time, which must be done to improve cardiorespiratory health and fitness. Cardiorespiratory health refers to the health of the heart, lungs, and blood vessels. It can be improved within a few weeks to a few months of regular physical activity. Three components of aerobic activity are intensity (how hard), duration (how long), and frequency (how often). Health benefits from physical activity have been shown to be gained at 150 minutes per week with the best results occurring when it is done across at least 3 days of the week (HHS, 2008).

Muscle-strengthening activities are another important component. Muscle-strengthening activity, or strength training, forces the body's muscles to work harder than normal. Strength training can be done through resistance training, lifting weights, supporting one's own body weight (i.e., push-ups, pull-ups, or lunges), or the use of bands. Strength training increases lean muscle mass, which raises the body's ability to use energy (HHS, 2008). The more lean muscle mass a body has, the more efficiently it can burn calories (Mayo Clinic staff, 2009b). Muscle-strengthening activities should involve all large muscles: legs, arms, back, chest, hips, abdomen, and shoulders. Muscle-strengthening activities also improve endurance, increase bone mass to help fight osteoporosis (the weakening of bones), and help to decrease recovery time from injury, trauma, or surgery (HHS, 2008). Bone-strengthening activities, otherwise known as weight-bearing activities, aid bone strength and growth. Examples include jumping jacks, running, walking briskly, and weight lifting (HHS, 2008).

Recommended Levels of Physical Activity

The *2008 Physical Activity Guidelines for Americans* (HHS, 2008) recommend children and adolescents get 60 minutes or more of moderate- or vigorous-intensity physical activity daily with most of the 60 minutes being aerobic activity. Strength training should be part of the 60 minutes of activity on at least 3 days per week. Those 60 minutes should also include bone-strengthening physical activity on at least 3 days of the week. More examples of bone-strengthening activities are jumping rope, basketball, tennis, and hopping (HHS, 2008).

Physical activity guidelines for adults include at least 150 minutes a week of moderate-intensity or 75 minutes a week of vigorous-intensity aerobic physical activity or an equivalent combination of moderate- and vigorous-intensity activity. Examples of moderate-intensity activities are walking briskly (3 mph or faster), water aerobics, bicycling at less than 10 mph, doubles tennis, ballroom dancing, or general gardening. Vigorous-intensity activities include race walking, jogging or running, swimming laps, singles tennis, aerobic dancing, bicycling at 10 mph or faster, jumping rope, heavy gardening (digging, mulching, or hoeing), or hiking uphill with a backpack (HHS, 2008). For more health benefits, adults can increase their aerobic physical activity to 300 minutes per week of moderate-intensity or 150 minutes a week of vigorous-intensity activity. Guidelines for older adults recommend that adults who cannot complete 150 minutes of moderate-intensity aerobic activity per week do as much physical activity as the conditions they have allow. Adults with disabilities should get at least 150 minutes of moderate-intensity or 75 minutes a week of vigorous-intensity aerobic activity if they are able. Adults with chronic medical conditions should do as much physical activity as their abilities allow while under the care of their health-care provider (HHS, 2008).

Participating in physical activity for at least 30 minutes per day for 5 days per week can promote one's health. For those individuals who find it difficult to set aside 30 or more continuous minutes for it, research continues to indicate that physical activity, or exercise, generates health benefits even in short bursts of time (American College of Sports Medicine, 2007; HHS, 2008). Becoming more physically active benefits people whether they exercise for 30-60 continuous minutes on most days of the week or add more movement daily in 10-minute sessions. The American College of Sports Medicine (2007) suggests fitting in physical activity by completing moderate-intensity aerobic activity in 10-minute sessions 3 times per day for 5 days per week.

Becoming more active by using large muscle groups will produce health benefits, so adding any extra daily movement is a step in the right direction (American College of Sports Medicine, 2007). Ways to add more physical activity daily include but are not limited to the following: parking a car further away from a desired destination, riding a bike, walking a pet, walking with a friend or family member, taking the stairs, push-mowing a yard instead of using a riding mower, cleaning floors, dancing, playing basketball, jogging, washing a car, raking leaves, playing with children or friends, swimming, getting up to change the television channel, doing sit-ups, pushups, or lunges during television commercials, carrying groceries, or gardening (Donatelle, 2010).

Injury Risk Reduction During Physical Activity

The *2008 Physical Activity Guidelines for Americans* (HHS, 2008) state that physical activity is safe for most people, especially during moderate-intensity activities, and that the health benefits from physical activity outweigh the risks. Individuals who have chronic health conditions or who are overweight or obese should discuss their plan for physical activity with their health-care provider before beginning. In order to reduce injury risks, one should begin physical activity with a warm-up and end with a cool-down. Warm-ups allow for a gradual increase in workloads and requirements from the heart and lungs while cool-downs allow a gradual slowing of the heart and lung functions. A good example of a warm-up and cool-down is walking (HHS, 2008).

The most common types of injuries from physical activity are bone, joint, muscle, ligament, or tendon injuries. Overheating or dehydration may also occur and, rarely, heart attacks may take place. Adding 5-15 minutes of light- to moderate-intensity activity to a person's regular activity level has a low risk of injury and no risk of severe cardiac events. Three factors—age, level of fitness, and prior experience—are important to consider when deciding how to increase activity level. Regarding age, the younger a person is, the more likely they will be able to increase activity in small amounts each week or two, compared to an older adult who needs more time (2-4 weeks) to adapt to a new activity. In addition, individuals should gradually increase the amount of their physical activity over time, depending on their fitness level. Those who are inactive should progress more slowly than those who are already active on a regular basis. Prior experience with physical activity enables a person to know what rates of increase work or do not work in regards to injury (HHS, 2008).

Pregnancy and the postpartum time period are additional considerations when exercising. Evidence indicates very low risk for healthy women who participate in moderate-intensity physical activity during pregnancy and postpartum. Pregnant women should avoid any activity that involves lying on their backs after the first trimester or any activity that involves a high risk of falling or abdominal injury. Pregnant women should consult their health-care provider about the proper physical activity amounts for them (HHS, 2008). Recommendations by the U.S. Department of Health and Human Services (2008) state that healthy women who are not already physically active with moderate-intensity to vigorous-intensity aerobic physical activity should get at least 150 minutes of moderate-intensity aerobic activity per week during pregnancy and postpartum. Pregnant women who have been regularly involved in vigorous-intensity aerobic physical activity pre-pregnancy can continue their physical activity as long as their health-care provider is made aware of it.

For her experience with physical activity, or exercise, we interviewed Janet, a 28-year-old woman. Janet started running when she was about 18 years old. Back then, she was unhappy with her body. She had never worked out and felt like she had never done anything. Janet's boss at the time, an avid runner, inspired Janet to go out one day and run. That first day was difficult for Janet because she hadn't been a runner before. She had to stop often and catch her breath. Janet was sore the next day but felt like she had made a difference in her body and improved her mental health with just that one run. Ever since that first outing, she has continued running.

Janet built up her endurance for running by setting goals to gradually go further and longer and achieving them. She then added gym workouts to her routine. Janet lifted weights and used machines like a stair master or treadmill. She also began practicing yoga. Janet experimented with different physical activities to avoid boredom. She's notices that, if she doesn't have a lot of time to work out, she becomes depressed, and running or working out does make her feel better. Keeping in shape and feeling good about her body also motivates Janet to continue her physical activity. In addition, she likens her time exercising to meditation, time to reflect with no distraction.

Janet's physically active lifestyle was once altered by a move to another state, which involved various factors, including cold weather. She stopped working out during that time, ate poorly, gained weight, and felt awful about herself. But, when the weather became warmer, she returned to her exercise routine, reaping all the noticeable benefits again. Another challenge to her physical activity has been arthritis in her lower body, which occasionally doesn't allow her to exercise. Also, staying with her routine and meeting her changing goals, which includes exercise classes, can be difficult for her to maintain. To others, Janet recommends not giving up. It took time for her to increase her endurance and ability and see changes in her body. She suggests adhering to and making time for a routine. Janet also advocates experimenting with different physical activities and being sure to make it fun, like by listening to music as she does during her workouts.

We interviewed Elizabeth, a 28-year-old woman, for her approach to physical activity, or exercise. Over a year before the interview, Elizabeth had begun to workout with a friend in a high school gym. She had recently ended a relationship with her boyfriend and wished to lose weight and become more toned. Elizabeth lifted weights and did cardio. She started with three times per week at that gym but grew unsatisfied with the schedule and that her friend was not always able to meet her. That led her to a local gym membership and going five times per week.

The challenges Elizabeth faced with her new lifestyle were allocating enough time for her exercise routine and motivating herself to go do it. Her mindset had to change. Elizabeth had to sacrifice other parts of her life for exercise and not let time conflicts leave it short because she realized that exercise increased her energy and happiness inward and out. Another difficulty was some feelings of animosity toward her for wanting to change and improve herself.

Elizabeth now feels better about herself and has more self-confidence because of her new healthier habits and mental approach. She has lost about 30 lbs and has gained overall muscle definition. Elizabeth's diet has changed remarkably as well. She knows it needed the transformation. She has left mayonnaise-laden potato chips for fruits and vegetables, and she passes on sugary foods. She also drinks the recommended amount of water and uses less alcohol and cigarettes.

Elizabeth realizes she spends more time in the gym than many others and is almost addicted to going, but she recommends going no matter how tired one is. She notes, instead of feeling it is required, a desire to be at the gym must exist and that she is now proud of her body. Elizabeth jokes that, prior to her current love for exercise, the only thing her old self ran for was the ice cream truck.

Conclusion

Physical activity promotes the health of those who participate in it regularly, and the physical and mental benefits from it can occur at any point in one's life. The health benefits for youth and adolescents from the recommended amounts include improved cardiorespiratory and muscle fitness, improved bone health, improved cardiovascular and metabolic health biomarkers, favorable body composition, and reduced symptoms of depression (HHS, 2008). Benefits for adults include lower risk for many health issues, including early death and coronary heart disease; lower risk for colon, breast, lung, and endometrial cancer; improved cardiorespiratory fitness and muscular fitness; better cognitive function and better functional health; and improved sleep quality (HHS, 2008). Regular physical activity produces health benefits starting in childhood and throughout a lifespan. Individuals that adopt physical activity into their lifestyles can increase their longevity, quality of life, and healthy years.

Recommendations

The following recommendations for safe physical activity are from the U.S. Department of Health and Human Services' *2008 Physical Activity Guidelines for Americans* (p. 36):

> To do physical activity safely and reduce risk of injuries and other adverse events, people should:
> - Understand the risks and yet be confident that physical activity is safe for almost everyone.
> - Choose to do types of physical activity that are appropriate for their current fitness level and health goals, because some activities are safer than others.
> - Increase physical activity gradually over time whenever more activity is necessary to meet guidelines or health goals. Inactive people should "start low and go slow" by gradually increasing how often and how long activities are done.
> - Protect themselves by using appropriate gear and sports equipment, looking for safe environments, following rules and policies, and making sensible choices about when, where, and how to be active.
> - Be under the care of a health-care provider if they have chronic conditions or symptoms. People with chronic conditions and symptoms should consult their health-care provider about the types and amounts of activity that are appropriate for them.

Selected Resources

American Academy of Pediatrics
141 Northwest Point Boulevard
Elk Grove Village, IL 60007
847-434-4000
www.aap.org/

American College of Sports Medicine
401 West Michigan Street
Indianapolis, IN 46202
317-637-9200
www.acsm.org/

Centers for Disease Control and Prevention
1600 Clifton Road
Atlanta, GA 30333
800-232-4636
www.cdc.gov/physicalactivity/index.html

National Institutes of Health
31 Center Drive, MSC 2292
Bethesda, MD 20892
800-222-4225
www.nia.nih.gov/HealthInformation/Publications/ExerciseGuide/

References

American Academy of Pediatrics. (2006). Active healthy living: Prevention of childhood obesity through increased physical activity. *Pediatrics, 117*(5), 1834-1842.

American College of Sports Medicine. (2007). *Physical activity & public health guidelines: Guidelines for healthy adults under age 65 - Tips for meeting the guidelines.* Retrieved February 22, 2011, from http://www.acsm.org/AM/Template.cfm?Section=Home_Page &TEMPLATE=CM/HTMLDisplay.cfm&CONTENTID=7764

American Diabetes Association. (n.d.). Food and fitness: Top 10 benefits of being active. Retrieved April 25, 2011, from http://www.diabetes.org/food-and-fitness/fitness/fitness-management/top-10-benefits-of-being.html

Centers for Disease Control and Prevention. (1997). Guidelines for school and community programs to promote lifelong physical activity among young people. *Morbidity and Mortality Weekly Report, 46*(No. RR-6).

Centers for Disease Control and Prevention. (2003). Prevalence of physical activity, including lifestyle among adults: United States, 2001-2002. *Morbidity and Mortality Weekly Report, 52*(32), 764-769.

Centers for Disease Control and Prevention. (2008). Prevalence of self-reported physically active adults – United States, 2007. *Morbidity and Mortality Weekly Report, 57*(48), 1297-1300.

Centers for Disease Control and Prevention. (2009a). FastStats:

Leading causes of death. Retrieved February 16, 2011, from http://www.cdc.gov/nchs/fastats/lcod.htm

Centers for Disease Control and Prevention. (2009b). Overweight and obesity: Economic consequences. Retrieved February 15, 2011, from http://www.cdc.gov/obesity/ causes/economics. html

Centers for Disease Control and Prevention. (2010a). Overweight and obesity: Defining overweight and obesity. Retrieved February 15, 2011, from http://www.cdc.gov/ obesity/defining. html

Centers for Disease Control and Prevention. (2010b). Vital signs: State-specific obesity prevalence among adults-United States, 2009. *Morbidity and Mortality Weekly Report, 59*(30), 951-955.

Centers for Disease Control and Prevention. (2011). Physical activity for everyone: Physical activity and health. Retrieved February 17, 2011, from http://www.cdc.gov/ physicalactivity/everyone/ health/index.html

Dalleck, L. C., & Kravitz, L. (2002). The history of fitness. *IDEA Health and Fitness Source, 20*(2), 26-33.

Daniels, S. R., Arnett, D. K., Eckel, R. H., Gidding, S. S., Hayman, L. L., Kumanyika, S., . . . Williams, C. L. (2005). Overweight in children and adolescents: Pathophysiology, consequences, prevention and treatment. *Circulation, 111*, 1999-2002.

Donatelle, R. J. (2010). *Health: The basics, Green edition.* San Francisco, CA: Pearson Education.

Finkelstein, E. A., Trogden, J. G., Cohen, J. W., & Dietz, W. (2009). Annual medical spending attributable to obesity: Payer- and service-specific estimates. *Health Affairs, 28*, 822-831.

Flegal, K. M., Carroll, M. D., Ogden, C. L., & Curtin, L. R. (2010). Prevalence and trends in obesity among US adults, 1999-2008. *Journal of the American Medical Association, 303*(3), 235-241.

Mayo Clinic staff. (2009a). Depression and anxiety: Exercise eases symptoms. Retrieved April 25, 2011, from http://www.mayoclinic.com/health/depression-and-exercise/MH00043

Mayo Clinic staff. (2009b). Metabolism and weight loss: How you burn calories. Retrieved February 22, 2011, from http://www.mayoclinic.com/health/metabolism/WT00006

Myers, J. (2003). Exercise and cardiovascular health. *Circulation, 107*, e2-e5.

Ogden, C. L., Carroll, M. D., Curtin, L. R., Lamb, M. M., & Flegal, K. M. (2010). Prevalence of high body mass index in U.S. children and adolescents, 2007-2008. *Journal of the American Medical Association, 303*(3), 242-249.

Thompson, D. L. (2011, March/April). Fitness focus copy-and-share: Exercise and diabetes. *ACSM's Health & Fitness Journal, 15*(2), 5.

U.S. Department of Health and Human Services. (1996). *Physical activity and health: A report from the Surgeon General.* Atlanta, GA: Author.

U.S. Department of Health and Human Services. (2008). *2008 Physical activity guidelines for Americans.* Retrieved from www.health.gov/paguidelines

U.S. Department of Health and Human Services. (2009). Physical activity and your heart: What is physical activity? Retrieved March 7, 2011, from http://www.nhlbi.nih.gov /health /dci/ Diseases/phys/phys_what.html

U.S. Department of Health and Human Services, Office of the

Surgeon General. (n.d.) Overweight and obesity: Health consequences. Retrieved February 19, 2011, from http://www.surgeongeneral.gov/topics/obesity/calltoaction/fact_consequences.html

U.S. Department of Health and Human Services, President's Council on Physical Fitness and Sports. (2000). *PCPFS research digests - Definitions: health, fitness, and physical activity.* Retrieved on March 7, 2011, from http://www.fitness.gov/digest_mar2000.htm

Warburton, D. E. R., Nicol, C. W., & Bredin, S. S. D. (2006, March 14). Health benefits of physical activity: The evidence. *Canadian Medical Association Journal, 174*(6), 801-809.

INJURY

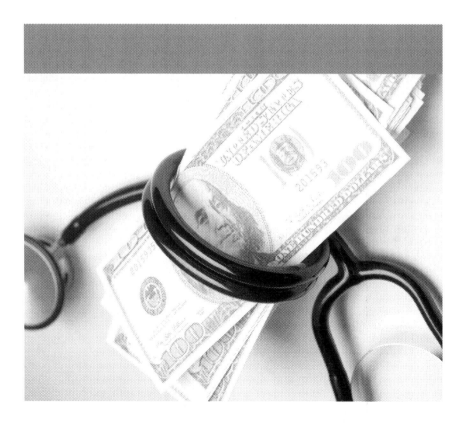

U nintentional injury is 1 of the 10 leading causes of death in the United States with 1 out of every 14 deaths caused by it (Bergen, Chen, Warner, & Fingerhut, 2008). Unintentional injuries are those injuries that occur without the intent for harm (Rice & MacKenzie, 1989). Unintentional injury includes homicide, falls, poisoning, motor vehicle accidents, violence, fire-related injuries, drowning, and more. With 7% of all deaths in the US resulting from unintentional injury, expenses top $400 billion in related lost work productivity and medical costs (Bergen et al., 2008). Unintentional injury affects all people regardless of age, race, and economic or educational level, and it can be prevented in many situations. The Centers for Disease Control and Prevention's National Center for Injury Prevention and Control (CDC, NCIPC, 2010a) reports that three fourths of all deaths among U.S. youth and adolescents are from unintentional injury. For teens 18-19 years of age, 4 out of every 5 deaths are due to it (CDC, NCIPC, 2010b), and it is the leading cause of death for people 1-44 years of age in the United States. For the aging population, falls lead the injury and death rates.

Sociocultural Influences

Injury prevention began as a focus in the U.S. workplace due to the high numbers of death and injury at work. In the 1800s, workplace safety was unheard of until Massachusetts passed the first safety legislation in 1887. By 1890, 21 states had followed suit by enacting health and safety legislation. The U.S. Department of

Labor initiated studies examining occupational safety and health issues in 1903. Dr. Alice Hamilton, known as the American founder of industrial medicine, spurred changes in occupational safety that eventually led to all states establishing work-related safety laws by the late 1930s. The Department of Labor created the Bureau of Labor Standards in 1934 which became the Occupational Health and Safety Administration (OSHA) in 1970.

Focus on safety outside the workplace began to evolve when consumer standards for health and safety improved as an offshoot to workplace standards (U.S. Department of Labor, Occupational Safety and Health Administration, 2009). In 1985, the National Research Council combined efforts with the Institute of Medicine (IOM) to address injury prevention outside the workplace and throughout the US. They recommended the Centers for Disease Control and Prevention (CDC) as the agency to best address injury prevention. In 1992, the CDC created the National Center for Injury Prevention and Control (the Injury Center), which concentrates on the consequences associated with injuries and violence as well as their prevention. The CDC's Injury Center gathers research and collects annual studies assessing injury and death in order to determine focus areas for nationwide injury prevention and guide related activities on an annual basis (CDC, NCIPC, 2009a). As the focus on injury prevention grew, the CDC collaborated with other professionals in injury prevention to better address the topic. In 1997, the IOM stated that no one agency alone could be adequate in addressing this issue and recommended that several agencies work together to assist while allowing the CDC to be the central agency in determining the approach (CDC, NCIPC, 2009a). In 2005, it dedicated prevention and control efforts to three areas: child maltreatment prevention, motor vehicle safety, and older adult falls prevention (CDC, NCIPC, 2010b). In addition to the Injury Center's focal points, other aspects of violence, poisoning, motor vehicle accidents, fire, and falls will be discussed in this chapter.

Violence

Child Maltreatment

Child maltreatment is a dedicated prevention focus in order to curb violence. Child maltreatment is any type of abuse to a child less than 18 years of age by his or her parent, caregiver, teacher, coach, or clergyperson. Abuse can be defined by each state individually, but most states define abuse as neglect, physical abuse, psychological abuse, or sexual abuse (U.S. Department of Health and Human Services, Administration for Children and Families [HHS, ACF], 2010). The World Health Organization (WHO) Consultation on Child Abuse Prevention defined it as follows:

> Child abuse or maltreatment constitutes all forms of physical and/or emotional ill-treatment, sexual, neglect or negligent treatment or commercial or other exploitation, resulting in actual or potential harm to the child's health, survival, development or dignity in the context of a relationship of responsibility, trust or power. (as cited in WHO, 2002, p. 59)

In 2008, over 3.5 million U.S. children were involved in individual reports to Child Protective Services (CPS) for reasons associated with abuse. Close to 60% of the reports were sent to CPS by teachers, police officers, lawyers, and social services professionals. Reported children and families of abuse receive preventive training by CPS (HHS, ACF, 2010). More than 70% of the victims in these reports suffered neglect, while 16.1% suffered physical abuse, 9.1% sexual abuse, and 7.3% psychological maltreatment. Abused at the highest rate (21.7 children per 1,000) were children up to one year of age (HHS, ACF, 2010). More than 80% of the perpetrators of violence against children were parents, an overwhelming 90% of them being the biological parent(s) of the child or children. Other relatives were 6.5% of the perpetrators. The overall death rate for abuse of children is 2.33 per 100,000 children. In 2008, more than 1,700 children died from abuse or neglect (HHS, ACF, 2010).

The CDC works nationally and internationally to combat child maltreatment and injuries. Strategies currently in action are aimed at individual, community, and societal levels to decrease risk factors for child maltreatment and injuries and to increase buffers against those risk factors. Education at all levels of the family, including prenatal family education, is one approach in preventive efforts being utilized. Other preventive efforts include programs that work to strengthen families, increase public awareness and supportive communities, and increase preventive programs and evaluation of those programs in communities nationwide. The CDC works closely with international organizations, such as the World Health Organization, the United Nations Children's Fund, the Violence Prevention Alliance, and many others, to develop, implement, and evaluate violence prevention programming worldwide (CDC, NCIPC, 2010j).

Youth Violence

Violence among U.S. youth includes bullying, slapping, hitting, robbery, electronic aggression, and assault. The negative impact of youth violence ranges from emotional to physical damage all the way to community damage via increased healthcare costs, decreased property values, and disrupted social services. In 2007, 5,764 U.S. youth 10-24 years of age were murdered; in 2008, more than 656,000 were treated in emergency rooms (CDC, NCIPC, 2010k). In 2009, 31% of youth surveyed in grades 9-12 reported having been in a physical fight within 12 months of the survey; 17.5% reported having carried a weapon (gun, knife, or club) within 30 days of the survey; and 5.9% reported having carried a gun one or more days within 30 days of the survey (CDC, 2010) Violence can set in during two periods of time in a youth's life. Early onset is at puberty and late onset is during early adolescence. The younger individuals start behaving violently, especially by age 13, the more crimes and more serious the crimes are that they tend to commit. Conversely, most children who have behavior problems or who display aggressive behavior as young children are not serious offenders of violence as they grow older. Most violence begins in adolescence and ends as one transitions into adulthood. Intervention and prevention programs for youth violence have been shown to be effective. Successful programs involve a comprehensive approach that addresses individual and environmental factors of both the children and their families. The strategy and quality of program implementation are key factors in determining the success of the violence prevention program (HHS, n.d.).

As electronic media has boomed in U.S. culture, more and more youth find they are navigating life in an electronic world. Electronic media provides many benefits. Unfortunately, risks are also associated with it, especially within the youth population. One risk is *electronic aggression*. The CDC defines electronic aggression as

> any kind of aggression perpetrated through technology—any type of harassment or bullying (teasing, telling lies, making fun of someone, making rude or mean comments, spreading rumors, or making threatening or aggressive comments) that occurs through e-mail, a chat room, instant messaging, a website (including blogs), text messaging, or videos or pictures posted on websites or sent through cell phones. (as cited in David-Ferdon & Hertz, 2009, p. 3)

Face-to-face aggression is still more common (Williams & Guerra, 2007), but recent research suggests incidents of electronic aggression are increasing. A study conducted in 2005 showed that, of 1,500 youth internet users between 10-17 years old, 9% (129) reported bullying or harassment compared to 6% in 2000 (Wolack, Mitchell, & Finkelhor, 2007). Common sites of aggression are chat rooms, websites, email, text messaging, and instant messaging (Kowalski & Limber, 2007). Victims of electronic aggression report feeling unsafe at school and distressed about the aggression (Ybarra, West, & Leaf, 2007). No current data supports any preventive efforts of electronic aggression. More research must be done to unveil preventive strategies (David-Ferdon & Hertz, 2009).

Sexual Violence

Another form of violence in the US is sexual violence. It includes unwanted physical contact, sexual harassment, threats, peeping, and taking nude photos. When U.S. high school students were surveyed in 2007, 8% of 9th through 12th graders reported being forced to have sex, the majority of which were females (CDC, 2008). In the US, 1 out of every 6 women and 1 out of every 33 men will report a rape or attempted rape during their lifetime. During their college years, the statistic for women becomes 1 in every 4 (Tjaden & Thoennes, 2000). Most cases go unreported by victims due to a variety of complex reasons, including embarrassment and fear. Victims who report sexual violence are more likely to report they suffer from chronic pain, headaches, stomach problems, sexually transmitted diseases, anxiety, fear, and depression. They are also more likely to participate in negative health behaviors such as smoking tobacco, drinking alcohol, using drugs, and engaging in risky sexual behaviors (CDC, NCIPC, 2009c).

Elder Violence
Elder violence, violence against those 60 years of age or older by a caregiver, includes physical violence, sexual violence, emotional violence, neglect, abandonment, and financial manipulation or misuse. Little data has been collected on elder abuse, but in 1996 there were 551,000 reported incidents of elder abuse, neglect, or self-neglect in the US (National Center on Elder Abuse, 1998). Many cases of elder abuse are thought to go unreported due to the victim's fear of telling police, family, or friends of the abuse (CDC, NCIPC, 2010l).

Dahlberg and Krug (2002) purport violence prevention be addressed at the individual, societal, community, and relationship levels throughout a lifespan, taking into account factors that may increase or decrease the likelihood of violence. Prevention strategies may include addressing attitude, knowledge, belief, cultural norms, policies, school and community practices, economic diversity, and more. The main goal of this social-ecological model is to, over a lifetime, change culture to one where positive health behaviors are attained and maintained (Dahlberg & Krug, 2002).

Unintentional Poisoning

According to the CDC, unintentional poisoning takes the lives of 75 people every day in the US and results in more than $26 billion in medical costs. Men carry a greater risk of unintentional poisoning than women and account for more than 70% of the medical costs for it on an annual basis. In 2008, over 700,000 emergency room visits were due to unintentional poisoning. Unintentional poisoning includes any non-purposeful overdose of recreational, over-the-counter, or prescription drugs as well as any excessive use of a drug or chemical by a toddler or child for non-recreational purposes (CDC, NCIPC, 2010m). Unintentional poisoning fatalities are highest in 35-54 year olds. For this age group, unintentional poisoning is the leading cause of death over motor vehicle accidents.

Prescription drugs, such as opioid pain medications, are of special concern with unintentional poisoning (Warner, Chen, & Makuc, 2009). Opioid pain medications have been prescribed at an increased rate due to their excellent ability to control pain. Between the years 1997 and 2007, cocaine and heroin followed opioids in unintentional poisoning fatalities (CDC, NCIPC, 2010m). Current recommendations for healthcare providers prescribing opioids for pain management include prescribing them only after non-opioid therapies do not work, using the lowest dose possible, considering drug testing in noncancer patients who have been on opioid medicines for longer than 6 weeks, and reporting to state prescription drug monitoring programs (CDC, NCIPC, 2010m).

While concern about prescription drug poisoning is on the rise, concern also exists for unintentional poisoning among children, which occurs frequently and is also preventable. It affected 71,000 children under the age of 17 between 2004 and 2005 (CDC, NCIPC, 2010f). Children are most likely to be poisoned from household products such as cleaning agents or chemicals (Schillie, Shehab, Thomas, & Budnitz, 2009). Recommendations to decrease unintentional poisonings include keeping household chemicals stored properly and out of reach of children, wearing protective clothing when working with chemicals, keeping fresh air a constant when working with chemicals, reading all directions in proper handling of chemicals, supervising children, keeping poisonous plants out of reach of children, and having the poison control phone number saved to a cell phone or near the home phone (CDC, NCIPC, 2011).

Falls

Falls account for preventable injury and death for both the young and old. Of the more than 9 million emergency room visits by children annually, more than 2 million were for injuries from falls (CDC, NCIPC, 2009b). For children 14 and younger, falls from playground equipment cost more than $1.5 million dollars in medical costs annually. Almost half of all playground injuries are severe fractures, amputations, internal injuries, concussions, and dislocations, with females sustaining these injuries at a higher rate than males (Tinsworth & McDonald, 2001). Properly maintained playgrounds, soft landing surfaces, and proper supervision can decrease the risk of falls from playground equipment (U.S. Consumer Product Safety Commission, n.d.).

Falls among older adults were responsible for 2.1 million hospital visits in 2008 (CDC, NCIPC, 2010b). Falls are the leading cause of injury in older adults, costing $19 billion in the year 2000 (CDC, NCIPC, 2010c). Among the population 65 and older, the cost of injuries from falls is expected to reach $32.4 million annually by 2020 (Englander, Hodson &, Terregrossa, 1996). As individuals age, their risk of falling increases. The most common injuries from falls in the population 65 and older are fractures of the spine, hip, pelvis, ankle, leg, or forearm (Scott, 1990). Traumatic brain injury (TBI), another common injury from falls, causes 46% of the fatalities from falls in older Americans (Stevens, 2006). Head injury and TBI have gained attention since brain imaging techniques have improved. Annually, 52,000 Americans die from TBI. The leading cause of brain injury for 0-4 year olds and the population 75 and older comes from falls. Motor vehicle injury is the leading cause of TBI in the 20-24 year-old age group. TBI affects 1.7 million Americans annually with males suffering the injury more often than females (Faul, Xu, Wald, & Coronado, 2010).

Traffic-Related Injuries and Death

The leading cause of unintentional injury fatalities is motor-vehicle-related crashes (Task Force on Community Preventive Services, 2001). Annually, motor-vehicle-related deaths and injuries cost the United States $500 for every licensed citizen, topping $97 billion, which is 2.0%-2.3% of the U.S. Gross National Product (Naumann, Dellinger, Zaloshnja, Lawrence, & Miller, 2010). In 2005, motor-vehicle-related injuries and deaths totaled 71% of the total costs for all fatal and non-fatal injuries in the US (Naumann et al., 2010).

Motor-vehicle-related fatal and non-fatal injuries in children 1-14 years of age most often occur via bicycle use without a helmet. These injuries and fatalities topped $7 billion in costs (Naumann et al., 2010). A simple preventative measure for this type of injury and cost would be to wear a helmet when bicycling. With helmet use, head injury risk during a crash is reduced by 60%, brain injury by 58% (Attewell, Glase, & McFadden, 2001). Laws requiring the use of helmets would increase the likelihood of bicyclists wearing them and could decrease the cost of injury and fatalities associated with bicycle use by at least $500 million (Naumann et al., 2010).

In 2006, over 30,000 fatalities and over 2 million injuries occurred to occupants in motor-vehicle crashes in the US (National Highway Traffic Safety Administration [NHTSA], 2008). The use of child safety seats and seat belts could greatly reduce these numbers. According to the Task Force on Community Preventive Services (2001) increasing child safety seat use in the US would raise infant safety in motor vehicle accidents by 70%, 47%-54% for children 1-4 years of age in relation to death, and decrease hospitalization by 69% for youth 4 years of age and younger. Seat belts worn properly with shoulder and lap belt have also been shown to be effective in decreasing death and severity of injury in motor vehicle crashes. When occupants were wearing lap and shoulder belts, deaths were reduced by 45%-60% and severe injuries to the head, chest, and extremities by 50%-83% (NHTSA, 1999). Enforcement and education related to wearing seat belts are valuable tools in decreasing injury and death rates as well as costs.

Another strategy set forth by the Task Force for Community Preventive Services (2001) to lower death and injury rates is to reduce alcohol-impaired driving. According to the CDC, 32 people in the US die daily from alcohol-impaired driving (CDC, NCIPC, 2010g). In 2008, about one third of all traffic-related fatalities occurred because of an alcohol-impaired driver. Alcohol-impaired drivers exist in all age groups. According to data collected by the CDC on an annual basis, in 2008 individuals 21-24 years of age were most likely to be driving under the influence of alcohol (34%), followed by 25-34 year olds (31%) and 35-44 year olds (25%). Fatalities where the driver had a BAC of .08% or higher were more likely to be a repeat offender (having been charged previously) for driving while intoxicated (CDC, NCIPC, 2010g). In addition to increased enforcement for alcohol-impaired driving, suggestions to decrease injury and fatalities related to alcohol-impaired driving include lowering the illegal BAC while driving to .05%, increasing taxes associated with alcohol, and increasing BAC testing at crash sites. Measures currently shown to be effective are sobriety checkpoints, community-based programming, health-promotion efforts, driver's license revoking, aggressive enforcement of .08% BAC laws, mandatory substance abuse treatment for offenders, and zero tolerance for driving under the influence of alcohol when under 21 years of age (CDC, NCIPC, 2010g).

Fire-Related Injury and Death

For fatal injuries suffered in U.S. homes, fires are the third leading killer (Runyan & Casteel, 2004). In 2009, not including firefighters, more than 2,500 people lost their lives to home fires and 13,000 were injured (Karter, 2010). Home fires cost $7.5 billion annually in medical costs alone (Finkelstein et al. 2006), and the majority of these fires occur during the winter months. Those 5 years or younger and those 65 or older represent a high risk for fatality in home fires when compared to the average person. Other risk factors include smoking, alcohol or drug use, disability, and not having smoke detectors installed in the home.

The leading cause of fire-related injuries is home cooking (Flynn, 2010). The leading cause of fire-related fatalities is smoking or smoking-related materials (Ahrens, 2010). Victims of fire from smoking-related material are less likely to be saved than victims of other fires (Hall, Ahrens, Rohr, Gamache, & Comoletti, 2006). According to the National Fire Protection Association (as cited in Hall, 2010) smoking-related material fires starting in living rooms, family rooms, dens, and bedrooms are the leading cause of fire-related deaths in the US, with one out of four victims not being the smoker themselves. Smoking-material fires start most frequently on mattresses and bedding, upholstered furniture, and trash. Between 1980 and 2008, fire-related deaths in the US decreased by 66% due to better safety regulations for mattresses and furniture as well as the overall decline in smokers (Hall, 2010).

Bill is a 51-year-old man who sustained life-threatening injuries from a bicycling accident. We asked him to describe his experience. The injuries occurred when he was cycling on a curvy road with a group of others and had to brake suddenly. Bill was thrown headfirst into an oncoming vehicle. He thanks his helmet for saving his life because he hit both sides of his head and cracked his skull. His back was also broken in two places and he suffered massive blood loss. After he was airlifted to a hospital, the doctors told Bill's wife it was unlikely he'd survive.

Bill made it through surgery, but, due to the accident, he permanently lost vision in one eye and hearing in one ear. And, at the time, whether he would ever walk again was in question. With Bill's severe head trauma, his doctor also didn't expect him to be able to go to school or work for at least five years. In addition, Bill had to be wary of becoming depressed because he faced numerous limitations and an overwhelming recovery process. Because of his brain injury, his doctors pushed him to read, learn new skills, and work on his damaged verbal ability. Bill also played a musical instrument and took music lessons as rehabilitation. Through therapy, he was able to start walking again.

After months in the hospital, he came home and for about another month required 24-hour supervision due to risk of seizure. He scheduled friends and family to be with him. He started walking more and more. Bill couldn't allow another brain injury, so he gave up bicycling, an activity he had enjoyed for over 30 years. His family did purchase a stationary bike for him to exercise on at home. Bill's healthy, athletic physical shape helped him through his recovery. For over a year, he also continued outpatient physical therapy and occupational therapy and saw a neuropsychologist. His medical bills and loss of income during his recovery did put a heavy strain on his family.

Due to his brain injury, Bill couldn't maintain his previous occupation of running a business, so he was encouraged to pursue another field and to have and create structure in his life. He started taking college classes one at a time, pushed himself in them, and began working again. He eventually applied to a university and was accepted. From his experience with recovery, he recommends trying to be present in every moment, moving methodically everyday, and working constructively with limitations and expectations. Bill's doctor told him it doesn't matter how well he does in any one day, session, or week of therapy; what matters is that he does a little bit everyday. Bill swears following this outlook changed his life for the better. Another approach that helped his recovery was a website a friend created that allowed Bill to communicate with people who supported him in his recovery, which made Bill feel loved and motivated to heal. They could see pictures, send gifts, or donate money as his medical bills mounted. Bill is very grateful to his family and friends for their tremendous support. At the time of the interview, just over five years after the accident, Bill was a few semesters away from graduating, a task many didn't think he could accomplish after his injuries.

For a unique angle on injury and its prevention, we interviewed Judy, a 36-year-old woman. Judy's awareness of issues with injury stems from some specific incidents in her past. Over 15 years ago, she was hit by a van traveling at 25-35 mph. The van's mirror struck and damaged her shoulder. Judy felt violated by that action and outraged by the police department's perceived acceptance of those types of collisions as common occurrences. A couple of months later, Judy totaled her car and sustained lower back injuries. She still has shoulder and back issues from those two incidents.

She decided not to purchase another car after that and, though she only suffered minor injuries, she had difficulty reconciling them. Judy's physical abilities were altered and she developed a fear of traffic. Those types of incidents and society's acceptance of them continued to trouble her. Her background led her to work in transportation and try to make her mark helping others in that arena.

Judy has suffered from other injuries in her lifetime as well. Each of her knees has been severely damaged from participating in sports. From those injuries, she has learned more about the mind-body connection and recommends not drowning in self-pity when injured but envisioning a full recovery and being active again. Meditating and imagining her body healing itself has helped her immensely. Her first knee injury was surgically repaired, but she allowed her second, very serious injury to her other knee to heal on its own, aided by positive meditation.

Judy has found that a yoga technique of imagining a channel of life energy and light filling her spine and healing has helped her with her injury. In addition, she has become a student of Reiki, a Japanese technique of promoting healing. She has also realized that posting her condition online opens the door to emotional and physical aid from many others and that having her status there makes the painful recounting of her injury unnecessary. Judy has learned from her injuries and has recognized that good can come from them.

Conclusion

Prevention of unintentional injury and death is a focus area in the CDC's Healthy People 2010 and 2020 initiatives. In August of 2007, leaders in unintentional injury and death prevention stated that 50 million people were injured in 2000 alone, costing the nation more than $400 billion in medical expenses. As unintentional injury continues to be a leading cause of death and injury in the United States, efforts at local, state, and national levels are continuing to be made in order to decrease the related pain, suffering, and costs (HHS, 2007). And everyone can take steps to decrease risks associated with unintentional injury on the individual level.

Recommendations

This section includes recommendations to prevent injury and death from unintentional injuries. Prevention of child and elder maltreatment and violence involves employing health-care practitioners to help recognize the signs and symptoms of it in these populations (CDC, NCIPC, 2010a). Educating parents and early home visitation by social work professionals are also prevention strategies for child maltreatment (WHO, 2002). Further research on effective prevention techniques are needed for both child and elderly maltreatment.

CDC Injury Center (2010h) recommendations for prevention of motor-vehicle-related injuries and fatalities:
- wearing seat belts
- using proper car seats for infants, toddlers, and children
- applying defensive-driving practices
- no drug or alcohol use while driving
- keeping the mind and eyes on the road
- keeping the hands on the wheel
- no texting or talking on the phone while driving
- graduated licensing

CDC Injury Center (2011) tips to prevent poisoning in children:

- Store all medicines and household products up and away and out of sight in a childproof cabinet where a child cannot reach them.
- When you are taking or giving medicines or are using household products:
- Do not put your next dose on the counter or table where children can reach them—it only takes seconds for a child to get them.
- If you have to do something else while taking medicine, such as answer the phone, take any young children with you.
- Secure the child safety cap completely every time you use a medicine.
- After using them, do not leave medicines or household products out. As soon as you are done with them, put them away and out of sight in a childproof cabinet where a child cannot reach them.
- Be aware of any legal or illegal drugs that guests may bring into your home. Ask guests to store drugs where children cannot find them. Children can easily get into pillboxes, purses, backpacks, or coat pockets.

CDC Injury Center (2011) tips for drug and medicine safety:
- Follow directions on the label when you give or take medicines. Read all warning labels. Some medicines cannot be taken safely when you take other medicines or drink alcohol.
- Turn on a light when you give or take medicines at night so that you know you have the correct amount of the right medicine.
- Keep medicines in their original bottles or containers.
- Never share or sell your prescription drugs. Keep all prescription medicines (especially opioid pain medications, such as those containing methadone, hydrocodone, or oxycodone), over-the-counter medicines (including pain or

fever relievers and cough and cold medicines), vitamins and herbals in a safe place that can only be reached by people who take or give them.

- Monitor the use of medicines prescribed for children and teenagers, such as medicines for attention deficit disorder, or ADD.
- Dispose of unused, unneeded, or expired prescription drugs. Follow the federal guidelines for how to do this.

CDC Injury Center (2010d) fall prevention strategies for the 65-and-older population:

- Exercise regularly. It's important that the exercises focus on increasing leg strength and improving balance. Tai Chi programs are especially good.
- Review medication lists—both prescription and over-the counter—with your doctor or pharmacist to reduce side effects and interactions that may cause dizziness or drowsiness.
- Have annual eye exams to maximize vision.
- Increase home safety by reducing tripping hazards, adding grab bars and railings, and improving the lighting in the home.

Additional ways to lower hip fracture risk include:

- Getting adequate calcium and vitamin D in your diet.
- Undertaking a program of weight bearing exercise.
- Getting screened and treated for osteoporosis.

CDC Injury Center (2010i) fall protection strategies for parents:

Wear a helmet and make sure your children wear helmets when:

- Riding a bike, motorcycle, snowmobile, scooter, or all-terrain vehicle;

- Playing a contact sport, such as football, ice hockey, or boxing;
- Using in-line skates or riding a skateboard;
- Batting and running bases in baseball or softball;
- Riding a horse; or
- Skiing or snowboarding.

Make living areas safer for children by:
- Installing window guards to keep young children from falling out of open windows; and
- Using safety gates at the top and bottom of stairs when young children are around.
- Making sure the surface on your child's playground is made of shock-absorbing material, such as hardwood mulch or sand.

CDC Injury Center (2010e) prevention strategies for fire-related injury and death in the home:
- Never leave food unattended on a stove.
- Keep cooking areas free of flammable objects (such as potholders and towels).
- Avoid wearing clothes with long, loose-fitting sleeves when cooking.
- Never smoke in bed or leave burning cigarettes unattended.
- Do not empty smoldering ashes in a trash can, and keep ashtrays away from upholstered furniture and curtains.
- Never place portable space heaters near flammable materials (such as drapery).
- Keep all matches and lighters out of reach of children. Store them up high, preferably in a locked cabinet.
- Install smoke alarms on every floor of the home, including the basement, and particularly near rooms in which people sleep.
- Use long-life smoke alarms with lithium-powered batteries and hush buttons, which allow persons to stop false alarms

quickly. If long-life alarms are not available, use regular alarms, and replace the batteries annually.

- Test all smoke alarms every month to ensure they work properly.
- Devise a family fire escape plan and practice it every 6 months. In the plan, describe at least two different ways each family member can escape every room, and designate a safe place in front of the home for family members to meet after escaping a fire.
- If possible, install or retrofit fire sprinklers into home.

Selected Resources

Centers for Disease Control and Prevention
National Center for Injury Prevention and Control
1600 Clifton Road
Atlanta, GA 30333
800-232-4636
www.cdc.gov/injury/

National Fire Protection Association
1 Batterymarch Park
Quincy, MA 02169
800-344-3555
www.nfpa.org/

National Highway Traffic Safety Administration
1200 New Jersey Avenue, SE
Washington, DC 20590
888-327-4236
www.nhtsa.gov

References

Ahrens, M. (2010). *Home structure fires.* Quincy, MA: National Fire Protection Association.

Attewell, R. G., Glase, K., & McFadden, M. (2001). Bicycle helmet efficacy: A meta-analysis. *Accident Analysis and Prevention, 33,* 345-352.

Bergen, G., Chen, L. H., Warner, M., & Fingerhut, L. A. (2008). *Injury in the United States: 2007 chartbook.* Hyattsville, MD: National Center for Health Statistics.

Centers for Disease Control and Prevention. (2008). Youth Risk Behavior Surveillance—United States, 2007. *Morbidity and Mortality Weekly Report, 57*(SS-4), 1-136. Retrieved from www.cdc.gov/healthyyouth/yrbs

Centers for Disease Control and Prevention. (2010). Youth Risk Behavioral Surveillance—United States, 2009. *Morbidity and Mortality Weekly Report, 59*(SS-5).

Centers for Disease Control and Prevention, National Center for Injury Prevention and Control. (2009a). Injury prevention & control: About CDC's Injury Center. Retrieved April 5, 2011, from http://cdc.gov/injury/about/index.html

Centers for Disease Control and Prevention, National Center for Injury Prevention and Control. (2009b). Protect the ones you love: Child injuries are preventable - CDC childhood injury report. Retrieved February 22, 2011, from http://www.cdc.gov/safechild /Child_Injury_Data.html

Centers for Disease Control and Prevention, National Center for

Injury Prevention and Control. (2009c). *Understanding sexual violence: Fact sheet, 2009.* Retrieved from http://cdc.gov/violenceprevention/pdf/SV_factsheet-a.pdf

Centers for Disease Control and Prevention, National Center for Injury Prevention and Control. (2010a). Injury Center: Violence Prevention - Elder maltreatment: Prevention strategies. Retrieved April 14, 2011, from http://www.cdc.gov/ViolencePrevention / eldermaltreatment/prevention.html

Centers for Disease Control and Prevention, National Center for Injury Prevention and Control. (2010b). Injury prevention & control: The burden of injury and violence: A pressing public health concern. Retrieved December 3, 2010, from http://www. cdc.gov/injury /overview/index.html

Centers for Disease Control and Prevention, National Center for Injury Prevention and Control. (2010c). Injury prevention & control: Home and recreational safety - Costs of falls among older adults. Retrieved November 18, 2010, from http://www. cdc.gov/ HomeandRecreationalSafety/Falls/fallcost.html

Centers for Disease Control and Prevention, National Center for Injury Prevention and Control. (2010d). Injury prevention & control: Home and recreational safety - Falls among older adults: An Overview. Retrieved November 30, 2010, from http://www. cdc.gov /HomeandRecreationalSafety/Falls/adultfalls.html

Centers for Disease Control and Prevention, National Center for Injury Prevention and Control. (2010e). Injury prevention & control: Home and recreational safety - Fire deaths and injuries: Prevention tips. Retrieved December 3, 2010, from http:// www.cdc.gov/HomeandRecreationalSafety/Fire-Prevention/ fireprevention.htm

Centers for Disease Control and Prevention, National Center for Injury Prevention and Control. (2010f). Injury prevention

& control: Home and recreational safety - Poisoning in the United States: Fact sheet. Retrieved November 30, 2010, from http://www.cdc.gov/HomeandRecreationalSafety/Poisoning/poisoning-factsheet.htm

Centers for Disease Control and Prevention, National Center for Injury Prevention and Control. (2010g). Injury prevention & control: Motor vehicle safety. Retrieved November 18, 2010, from http://www.cdc.gov/Motorvehiclesafety/index.html

Centers for Disease Control and Prevention, National Center for Injury Prevention and Control. (2010h). Injury prevention & control: Motor vehicle safety - Distracted driving. Retrieved April 14, 2011, from http://www.cdc.gov/Motorvehiclesafety/Distracted_Driving/index.html

Centers for Disease Control and Prevention, National Center for Injury Prevention and Control. (2010i). Injury prevention & control: Traumatic brain injury - Prevention. Retrieved April 14, 2011, from http://www.cdc.gov /traumaticbraininjury/prevention.html

Centers for Disease Control and Prevention, National Center for Injury Prevention and Control. (2010j). Injury prevention & control: Violence prevention - Global violence prevention. Retrieved November 28, 2010, from http://www.cdc.gov/ViolencePrevention /globalviolence/index.html

Centers for Disease Control and Prevention, National Center for Injury Prevention and Control. (2010k). *Understanding youth violence: Fact sheet, 2010*. Retrieved from http://www.cdc.gov/violenceprevention/pdf/YV-FactSheet-a.pdf

Centers for Disease Control and Prevention, National Center for Injury Prevention and Control. (2010l). *Understanding elder maltreatment: Fact sheet, 2010*. Retrieved from http://www.cdc.gov/violenceprevention/pdf/EM-FactSheet-a.pdf

Centers for Disease Control and Prevention, National Center for Injury Prevention and Control. (2010m). *Unintentional drug poisoning in the United States.* Retrieved from http://www.cdc. gov/HomeandRecreationalSafety/pdf/poison-issue-brief.pdf

Centers for Disease Control and Prevention, National Center for Injury Prevention and Control. (2011). Injury prevention & control: Home and recreational safety - Tips to prevent poisonings. Retrieved December 1, 2010, from http://www.cdc. gov/ HomeandRecreationalSafety/Poisoning/preventiontips. htm

Dahlberg LL, Krug EG. Violence-a global public health problem. In: Krug E, Dahlberg LL, Mercy JA, Zwi AB, Lozano R, eds. World Report on Violence and Health. Geneva, Switzerland: World Health Organization; 2002:1–56

David-Ferdon, C., & Hertz, M. F. (2009). *Electronic media and youth violence: A CDC issue brief for researchers.* Atlanta, GA: Centers for Disease Control and Prevention.

Englander, F., Hodson, T. J., & Terregrossa, R. A. (1996). Economic dimensions of slip and fall injuries. *Journal of Forensic Science, 41*(5), 733-746.

Faul, M., Xu, L., Wald, M. M., & Coronado, V. G. (2010). *Traumatic brain injury in the United States: Emergency department visits, hospitalizations and deaths 2002–2006.* Atlanta, GA: Centers for Disease Control and Prevention, National Center for Injury Prevention and Control.

Finkelstein EA, Corso PS, Miller TR, Associates. Incidence and Economic Burden of Injuries in the United States. New York: Oxford University Press; 2006.

Flynn, J. D. (2010). *Characteristics of home fire victims.* Quincy, MA: National Fire Protection Association.

Hall, J. R., Jr. (2010). *The smoking-material fire problem* (NFPA No. USS10). Retrieved from http://www.nfpa.org/assets/files/PDF/OS.Smoking.pdf

Hall, J. R., Jr., Ahrens, M., Rohr, K., Gamache, S., & Comoletti, J. (2006). *Behavioral mitigation of smoking fires through strategies based on statistical analysis.* Retrieved from http://www.usfa.dhs.gov/downloads/pdf/publications/fa-302-508.pdf

Karter, M. J. (2010). *Fire loss in the United States during 2009.* Quincy, MA: National Fire Protection Association, Fire Analysis and Research Division.

Kowalski, R. M., & Limber, S. P. (2007). Electronic bullying among middle school students. *Journal of Adolescent Health, 41*(Suppl.), S22-S30.

National Center on Elder Abuse. (1998). *National elder abuse incidence study: Final report.* Washington, DC: American Public Human Services Association.

National Highway Traffic Safety Administration. (1999). *Fourth report to Congress: Effectiveness of occupant protection systems and their use* (DOT HS 808 919). Washington, DC: U.S. Department of Transportation, National Highway Traffic Safety Administration.

National Highway Traffic Safety Administration. (2008). *2006 Motor vehicle occupant protection facts* (DOT HS 810 654; Reprinted August 2008). Retrieved from http://www.nhtsa.gov/DOT/NHTSA/Traffic%20Injury%20Control/Articles / Associated%20Files/810654.pdf

Naumann, R. B., Dellinger, A. M., Zaloshnja, E., Lawrence, B. A., & Miller, T. R. (2010). Incidence and total lifetime costs of motor vehicle–related fatal and nonfatal injury by road user type, United States, 2005. *Traffic Injury Prevention, 11*(4), 353-360.

Rice, D. & MacKenzie, E. (1989). *Cost of injury to the United States: A report to congress.* San Francisco, CA: Institute for Health & Aging, University of California and Injury Prevention Center, The Johns Hopkins University.

Runyan, S. W., & Casteel, C. (Eds.). (2004). *The state of home safety in America: Facts about unintentional injuries in the home* (2nd ed.). Washington, DC: Home Safety Council.

Schillie, S. F., Shehab, N., Thomas, K. E., & Budnitz, D. S. (2009). Medication overdoses leading to emergency department visits among children. *American Journal of Preventive Medicine, 37*, 181-187.

Scott, J. C. (1990). Osteoporosis and hip fractures. *Rheumatic Disease Clinics of North America, 16*(3), 717-40.

Stevens, J. A. (2006). Fatalities and injuries from falls among older adults – United States, 1993–2003 and 2001–2005. *Morbidity and Mortality Weekly Report, 55*(45).

Task Force on Community Preventive Services. (2001). Recommendations to reduce injuries to motor vehicle occupants: Increasing child safety seat use, increasing safety belt use, and reducing alcohol-impaired driving. *American Journal of Preventive Medicine, 21*(4S), 16-22.

Tinsworth, D., & McDonald, J. (2001). *Special study: Injuries and deaths associated with children's playground equipment.* Washington, DC: U.S. Consumer Product Safety Commission.

Tjaden, P., & Thoennes, N. (2000). *Extent, nature, and consequences of intimate partner violence: Findings from the National*

Violence Against Women Survey (Publication No. NCJ 181867). Retrieved from www.ojp.usdoj.gov/nij/pubs-sum/181867.htm

U.S. Consumer Product Safety Commission. (n.d.). *Public playground safety checklist* (CPSC Document No. 327). Retrieved November 20, 2010, from http://www.cpsc.gov/cpscpub /pubs/327.html

U.S. Department of Health and Human Services. (n.d.). *Youth violence: A report of the Surgeon General.* Retrieved November 28, 2010, from http://www.surgeongeneral.gov/library/youthviolence/chapter1/sec1.html#intro

U.S. Department of Health and Human Services. (2007, August). *Injury and violence prevention.* Retrieved December 1, 2010, from http://www.healthypeople.gov/Data/2010prog/focus15/2007Focus15.pdf

U.S. Department of Health and Human Services, Administration for Children and Families, Administration on Children, Youth and Families, Children's Bureau. (2010). *Child Maltreatment 2008.* Retrieved from http://www.acf.hhs.gov/programs/cb / stats_research/index.htm#can

U.S. Department of Labor, Occupational Safety and Health Administration. (2009). *Reflections on OSHA's History* (OSHA 3360). Retrieved from http://www.osha.gov/history /OSHA_HISTORY_3360s.pdf

Warner, M., Chen, L. H., & Makuc, D. M. (2009). *Increase in fatal poisonings involving opioid analgesics in the United States, 1999–2006* (NCHS Data Brief No. 22). Hyattsville, MD: National Center for Health Statistics.

Williams, K. R., & Guerra, N. G. (2007). Prevalence and predictors of internet bullying. *Journal of Adolescent Health, 41*(Suppl.), S14-S21.

Wolak, J., Mitchell, K. J., & Finkelhor, D. (2007). Does on-line harassment constitute bullying? An exploration of online harassment by known peers and online only contacts. *Journal of Adolescent Health, 41*(Suppl.), S51-S58.

World Health Organization. (2002). Child abuse and neglect by parents and othercaregivers. In *World report on violence and health* (pp. 57-86). Retrieved from http://www.who.int / violence_injury_prevention/violence/global_campaign/en/chap3.pdf

World Health Organization. (2010). Disability, injury prevention and rehabilitation. Retrieved November 28, 2010, from http://www.searo.who.int/en/Section1174/Section1461.htm

Ybarra, M., West, M. D., & Leaf, P. (2007). Examining the overlap in internet harassment and school bullying: Implications for school intervention. *Journal of Adolescent Health, 41*(Suppl.), S42-S50.

SEXUAL HEALTH

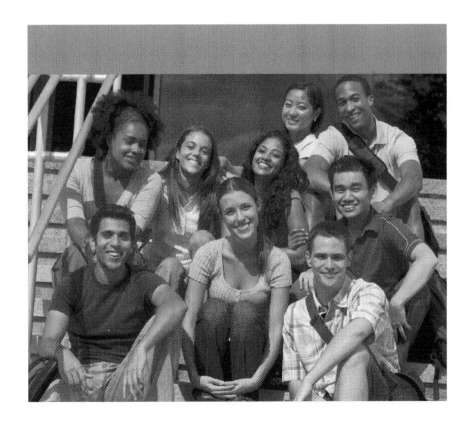

The World Health Organization defines sexual health as mental, physical, social, and emotional well-being in relation to sexuality along with the absence of disease, dysfunction, violence, coercion, or discrimination while maintaining sexual rights and respect (as cited in American Social Health Association [ASHA], 2010i). Sexual health includes knowing when sexual activity is appropriate and being able to communicate with a partner about personal needs whether they involve sexual activity or not. Sexual health also includes parents educating their children about emotions, intimacy, moral values, personal responsibility, sexual orientation, gender differences, and self image (ASHA, 2010h). Sexual health involves communication, education, and a clear understanding of disease prevention. This chapter focuses on disease prevention.

Sociocultural Influences on Sexually Transmitted Diseases

Adult-focused discussion of sexually transmitted diseases (STDs) dates back to Europe in the 15th century. In the US during the 18th century, STDs were referred to as *venereal diseases* and were thought to exist due to prostitution and new immigrants with less moral fiber than previous immigrants (Sacco, 2004). In the 19th and 20th centuries, individuals in the US found to be infected with a venereal disease were thought of as cruel individuals lacking moral depth. Infection was legitimate reason for divorce. Overwhelmingly, the fault for infection was placed upon women. No accurate count or treatment of venereal disease existed during this time and most accounts referred only to syphilis (Adler, 1980). It was not until the discovery of penicillin in the 1940s that a treatment was available. Research and treatment in the field continue to grow today (Sacco, 2004).

During the last 25 years, the field of sexual health has experienced important growth in knowledge and technology, allowing for better informed individuals (Pan American Health Organization & World Health Organization, 2000). The CDC currently collects yearly statistics on STDs based on information from state health departments nationwide. This information is used to help create prevention information to disseminate in order to decrease the rate of STDs in the US. With 19 million new diagnoses of STDs annually, about half occurring in 15-24 year olds (ASHA, 2010g), and it all costing an estimated $16.4 billion each year, prevention of disease is a major focus in sexual health (CDC, 2010a).

Sexually Transmitted Infections

Sexually transmitted disease and *sexually transmitted infection* are terms that can be used interchangeably. STDs are viral or bacterial infections transmitted through sexual activity (anal, oral, or vaginal sex and in some cases skin-to-skin contact). Many different types of STDs exist, some of which are curable while others are symptom treatable. Some viral and bacterial STDs will present with symptoms (symptomatic) in an infected person while others will not (asymptomatic). In recent years, testing, education, treatment, and availability of treatment have all improved. A nationwide increase in reported STDs is most likely from an increase in screening for them, more sensitive STD testing, and a better state-level system to report STDs to the CDC.

Diagnosis of STDs is important because some untreated STDs can cause complications with fertility as with pelvic inflammatory disease (PID). In addition, having an STD can increase the likelihood of transmitting human immunodeficiency virus, or HIV (CDC, 2010a). Viral STDs can be treated by attempting to control the symptoms or by vaccinating against the virus prior to risky behaviors, but currently no cure for viral STDs exists. Bacterial STDs can be treated with antibiotics and cured, and it is important that individuals infected with a bacterial STD tell their sexual partners to get checked. If only one partner receives antibiotic treatment for a bacterial STD, he or she will likely get the infection back from the untreated partner. Any person who has been sexually active with an infected person should be tested for STDs, so they may also receive treatment (CDC, 2010a).

Common STDs

Chlamydia. Chlamydia is the most common bacterial STD in the US. In 2009, more cases of chlamydia than ever were reported to the CDC. For every 100,000 people in the US, there were 409.2 reported cases of chlamydia, which affected women at a greater rate than men (CDC, 2010a). Infected males may note burning or itching around the opening of the penis, pain during urination, or discharge from the penis. Untreated infection in males can cause damage to the epididymis leading to pain, fever, and occasionally infertility. Chlamydia produces little or no symptoms in women and can be passed on to a fetus during delivery. Most women will have no symptoms when infected. If a woman does present symptoms, she will within one to three weeks of infection. Early symptoms include abnormal vaginal discharge and/or pain during urination. If the infection goes untreated and travels into the reproductive tract, women may experience no symptoms at all or may report lower back or abdominal pain, pain during intercourse, or abnormal menstrual bleeding and may also encounter pelvic inflammatory disease (PID). PID causes damage and inflammation to the fallopian tubes, uterus, and surrounding tissue. For 10%-15% of women who go untreated for chlamydia, infertility or ectopic pregnancies are the result (CDC, 2010b). Recommendations for chlamydia screening include yearly testing for all sexually active women under the age of 25, all pregnant women, and any older woman who has multiple sex partners or a new sex partner. It is possible to contract a chlamydia infection of the rectum during anal intercourse or of the throat during oral sex. Symptoms of a chlamydia infection of the rectum include rectal pain, discharge, and bleeding.

Gonorrhea. Gonorrhea is a bacterial STD that can be cured with antibiotics. As of 2008-2009, gonorrhea occurs in about 99 of every 100,000 people. The highest rates of gonorrhea are found in the age groups of 15-19 and 20-24 years of age (CDC, 2010a). The bacterium that causes gonorrhea can grow in the uterus, cervix, fallopian tubes, urethra, mouth, throat, eyes, and anus (CDC, 2010d). As with chlamydia, gonorrhea may produce no symptoms in males or females. If symptoms appear, they will within 2-30 days of infection transmission. Symptoms of infection in males include pain during urination, yellow, green, or white discharge from the penis, and occasional painful or swollen testes. The majority of infected females will have no symptoms at all. If a female has symptoms, they are painful urination, abnormal discharge, and bleeding between periods (CDC, 2010d). PID is also a concern for untreated gonorrhea. Untreated infection in a pregnant woman can cause serious complications for the fetus during development or the baby during delivery. In males, the epididymis can become inflamed, causing infertility issues (CDC, 2010d).

Herpes. Herpes is a virus that can cause sores on the mouth, genitals, or rectum. Transmission occurs from vaginal, anal, or oral sex. Females are more likely to become infected by their male partner than a male becoming infected by his female partner. The two types of herpes are herpes simplex virus 1 (HSV-1) and herpes simplex virus 2 (HSV-2). HSV-1 tends to prefer the site around the mouth, causing an outbreak of fluid-filled blisters that carry the virus. The fluid-filled blisters then become sores until healed. It is possible for oral herpes, HSV-1, to be transmitted to another person's genitals through oral-genital or genital-genital contact. HSV-2 also causes fluid filled blisters; however, this virus prefers the area of the genitals or rectum. HSV-2 can also be transmitted to another person by oral-genital or genital-genital contact. In addition, it is possible for both types of the virus to be left on the skin of an infected person and then be transmitted to a partner's skin (CDC, 2010c). Approximately 1 in 6 people between 14 to 49 years of age in the US have genital HSV-2, which affects women at a greater rate than men (CDC, 2010c).

In order to prevent transmission of herpes to another person, one should avoid sexual contact during an active outbreak of sores or fluid-filled blisters and use a condom during all sexual contact between outbreaks. When a person has no symptoms of herpes, it is still possible to transmit the virus to another person. This process is called *asymptomatic viral shedding* (ASHA, 2010a). A suppressive antiviral medication is also available to decrease the likelihood of transmission, severity, and number of outbreaks in infected individuals. Herpes can be spread to a baby during vaginal delivery. Mothers who are infected with herpes should discuss their options with their health-care provider (ASHA, 2010a). Persons infected with herpes are also more susceptible to contracting HIV (ASHA, 2010a).

Human Papilloma Virus (HPV). HPV is a virus that has approximately 100 strains, 30 of which can affect the genitals or cells of the cervix. The remaining strains of HPV can cause warts on the skin, such as on hands or feet (ASHA, 2010b). Rarely, the virus can cause warts in the mouth or throat. Also uncommon from HPV is cancer of the penis, vulva, vagina, anus, head, and neck, which includes the tongue, tonsils, and throat (CDC, 2009). Certain strains of the genital HPV virus can lead to cervical cancer. This type of cancer can be easily treated if women visit their healthcare provider for Pap smear screening, which would detect cervical changes before the cancer develops and allow for treatment. Cervical cancer takes years to develop (ASHA, 2010b).

Each year, about 6 million new cases of HPV occur in the US, while it is estimated that 20 million people have the virus at any given time. Many people are infected with HPV but have no warts, so they do not know they have the virus. The CDC states that in more than 90% of HPV cases, the body's own immune system will clear the infection within two years of contracting the virus. Sexual contact (vaginal, anal, oral) and skin-to-skin contact can transmit the virus, so it is recommended that latex or polyurethane condoms are used for each sex act from beginning to end. Other recommendations to prevent the infection include having a monogamous relationship, having few lifetime sex partners, abstinence, and vaccine. Two vaccines are currently on the market for HPV. One vaccine protects against four strains, two that cause genital warts and two that cause cervical cancer. Both vaccines are recommended for women ages 9-26 years. Currently, one vaccine is approved for use on men 9-26 years of age. Each brand of vaccine consists of three shots spread out over time. It is recommended a person have the same brand shot for all three shots in the vaccine series (CDC, 2009).

HIV/AIDS. HIV (human immunodeficiency virus) attacks the body's immune system. AIDS (acquired immune deficiency syndrome), which is caused by HIV, is a slow progressing life-threatening disease that occurs when the body's immune system can no longer fight infection due to a severe depletion in a person's white blood cells, or CD4 (Mayo Clinic staff, 2010). HIV can be transmitted through blood, breast milk, or sexual fluids, so it can spread via unprotected sexual contact with an infected partner; mother to baby during pregnancy, delivery, or breastfeeding; or with drug use by sharing needles or equipment with an infected person (ASHA, 2010d). The virus weakens the body's immune system over time. Opportunistic infections that would easily be handled by healthy immune systems can cause illness or even death in a person infected with HIV (ASHA, 2010d).

Recommended strategies to reduce the risk of contracting HIV include: abstinence; having a long-term monogamous, non-infected partner; using a latex or polyurethane condom during any act of sex (oral, anal, vaginal); using dental dams (during oral sex) or female condoms; delaying the age when sexual activity begins; reducing the number of sex partners a person has; practicing non-penetrative sex; and getting tested for STDs and encouraging a partner to be tested as well (ASHA, 2010e). Individuals infected with another STD are more susceptible to contracting or transmitting HIV, emphasizing the importance of treating STDs in all populations

(Fleming & Wasserheit, 1999). Techniques for HIV testing have evolved since the 1990s. Currently, blood tests and rapid tests are available. The tests look for antibodies that take at least three months and rarely up to six months to develop in an infected person from the time of contraction. Benefits of testing include being able to apply preventive treatments to stay healthy while living with the virus and decreasing the likelihood of transmitting the virus to another person. Many sites offer either confidential or anonymous HIV testing. Counseling is important if a person or partner is HIV positive (ASHA, 2010f).

Hepatitis. Hepatitis is a virus that causes inflammation of the liver and is the most common cause of liver cancer and liver transplants. Approximately 4.4 million Americans live with chronic hepatitis while 80,000 new infections occur each year. The populations most at risk of contracting hepatitis are men who have sex with men, intravenous drug users, those with HIV/AIDS, or those who already have an STD. There are many types of hepatitis, and they are transmitted in different ways. Hepatitis A can be transmitted during sexual activity via the fecal-oral route (CDC, 2010e). Hepatitis B is transmitted by blood, saliva, semen, or vaginal secretions (ASHA, 2010c). Rarely, hepatitis C can be transmitted via sexual activity but is more readily transmitted through contact with human blood, and its risk factors include multiple sex partners, other STDs, or sex trauma. Condoms work to lower the risk of transmission of hepatitis B and C. Hepatitis B and A have highly recommended vaccinations available to help prevent the disease (CDC, 2010e).

Trichomoniasis. Trichomoniasis is a sexually transmitted single cell protozoan with an estimated 7.4 million new cases in males and females annually. Women tend to have the infection at higher rates than men. Symptoms in men are often nonexistent; however, if symptoms do occur, they include irritation of the penis, mild discharge, and slight burning during urination or ejaculation. Women who have signs of the infection report frothy green and odorous discharge with pain during intercourse and or urination within 5-28 days of transmission (CDC, 2007). Pregnant women infected with trichomoniasis have premature or low birth weight babies. Treatment for trichomoniasis includes diagnosis by a health-care provider and prescription medication for both partners as re-infection is common among partners due to lack of symptoms. Untreated trichomoniasis can increase the likelihood of transmission of HIV to either partner. Prevention of the infection includes long-term monogamous relationships, latex condoms, and abstinence (CDC, 2007).

Treatment and Prevention

In 2005, the CDC convened with professionals from the STD field to discuss guidelines for treatment and prevention recommendations for the US (Workowski & Berman, 2006). Prevention guidelines focus on the health-care provider and emphasize the following: educating patients who are at risk in order to change their sexual behavior; identifying individuals who are asymptomatic with infection and those who are infected with symptoms yet unlikely to get screening or treatment for STDs; increasing diagnosis and treatment; evaluating, treating, and counseling partners of infected individuals; and increasing vaccinations for those who are not yet sexually active (Workowski & Berman, 2006).

Other methods of reducing STD transmission include abstinence or long-term monogamous relationships, pre-exposure vaccinations, condoms, and spermicides. Abstinence, which is abstaining from any sexual activity, is the most reliable way to ensure low to no risk of STD transmission. For those interested in pursuing long-term monogamous relationships, STD testing prior to sexual activity in the relationship is recommended for both partners. Pre-exposure vaccinations are vaccinations against viral STDs before sexual activity ever begins. Currently, there are vaccines for hepatitis A and B and human papillomavirus (HPV strains 6, 11, 16, & 18) and clinical trials looking for other viral STD vaccinations (Workowski & Berman, 2006). Spermicide studies have shown that spermicides are not effective in reducing STD transmission rates.

In addition, studies showed an increase in HIV transmission rates with frequent use of spermicides due to the breaking down of cell tissue by increased use of the product.

Condoms are available over the counter in forms for both males and females. The female condom, which is made of polyurethane, has had fewer studies done on it, but it has been shown to be effective in reducing the risk of STD transmission. The CDC recommends using this barrier method when condoms are not present. The male latex condom is effective in reducing the risk of STD transmission when used correctly. The male condom also comes in nonlatex forms, such as polyurethane or natural membrane condoms. Polyurethane condoms are effective in reducing the risk of pregnancy and STDs, but natural membrane condoms (sometimes called lambskin condoms) are not effective in reducing the risk of STD transmission (Workowski & Berman, 2006).

For insight into an individual's sexual health, we interviewed Sarah, a 26-year-old woman. Sarah grew up in a different country where sexual health education was an integral part of her schooling. She discussed sexual health with her friends from the time she was in elementary school through her university education, and now her studies include a research interest in sexuality.

Sarah feels her personal life has been impacted by her current research because her knowledge of sexuality may be intimidating to other people, but she ultimately feels that her knowledge can be to her benefit. She is more aware of the importance of maintaining a sexual well-being and how happiness from one's sexual and relationship life impacts other areas of life. She believes people do not recognize this and always tend to focus on the disease aspect of sexuality. Disease is only one part of sexual health. For her, sexual health includes sexual pleasure and satisfaction and relationship satisfaction, which carry over into being satisfied with the rest of one's life. Preventing disease is of initial concern, but a healthy mind in terms of sexuality is of more interest to her.

Sarah has not needed to deal with personal sexual health issues, though through her field of work, she sees many individuals with recurrent sexually transmitted infections or recurrent unwanted pregnancies. Sarah recognizes the difficulty they have in trying to change their behavior. She believes they need to want to change and realize that the cost outweighs any benefit before it is too late and, for example, they contract HIV. So, for her, it is important to prevent infection, but it is also imperative to pay attention to the psychological, cultural, and sociological influences that contribute to sexual well-being and sense of self. She believes that a more comprehensive sexual health education at a young age is extremely important and that it would limit much disease and unwanted pregnancy. Sarah recommends that individuals coping with a sexual health issue or those who are interested in such issues should be made aware of the wealth of reliable resources available and be able to find accurate information.

We interviewed Greg, a 26-year-old, for his perspective on sexual health. Greg became interested in studying sexual health when he was younger. He had a steady interest in HIV and AIDS then, but he was not sure whether he wanted to study their medical or social aspects. When Greg came out as an openly gay man, he recognized that he had become part of a community where HIV and AIDS have a history and sociopolitical ramifications. Greg has thought about gender, sexuality, identity, and public health in this context and has entered a program of study in sociology.

In his research, Greg finds the inherent focus on risky behaviors and protection challenging. He prefers to concentrate on the sociocultural aspects of the identity and behavior of gay men and how they regard themselves as both men and gay. Greg has been a part of HIV outreach organizations since beginning college, but what intrigues him personally is that even though he was well aware of how to protect himself, he did not always follow what he told others.

Greg believes that sexual health education should be centered on culturally specific strategies and informing people of the normality of sexual behaviors, even the atypical behaviors, which he also considers normal. For Greg, concentrating more on what is promoting the risky sexual behavior in sociocultural terms and how that aspect leads to outcomes of disease is needed in concert with the attention on the behaviors themselves.

Conclusion

Effective measures can reduce the rate of STDs in the US and worldwide. Bacterial STDs can now be treated and cured. In some cases, viral STDs can be controlled by vaccination or the body's own immune response. Other viral STDs can be better controlled with the use of anti-viral medications. Education on reducing the risk of transmitting or contracting an STD should also include both abstinence and prevention via condoms. STDs can be reduced by individuals utilizing condoms, but total abstinence is the only 100% effective measure in reducing a person's risk for STDs. Clear prevention messages and outreach to the public to make preventive practices a common behavior must continue. The combined efforts of scientists, medical professionals, agencies, and organizations have helped to make information that can decrease the spread of STDs available.

Recommendations

CDC (2011) recommendations to reduce the risk of STDs:

- Be abstinent (no kind of sexual activity).
- Be in a long-term mutually monogamous relationship where each partner has been STD tested and known to be uninfected.
- Yearly chlamydia testing among sexually active women 25 years or younger, older women with risk factors, and all pregnant women.
- If any unusual genital symptoms are present, stop having sex and consult a health care provider.
- Women and men who are told they have an STD should notify all of their recent sex partners (sex partners within

the preceding 60 days) so they can see a health care provider and be evaluated for an STD.
- Sexual activity should not resume until both partners have been examined and, if necessary, treated.
- If sexually active, latex condoms, when used correctly and consistently can reduce the risk of STDs.

Recommendations from Workowski and Berman (2006) for using a condom correctly:
- Use a new condom with each sex act (e.g., oral, vaginal, and anal).
- Carefully handle the condom to avoid damaging it with fingernails, teeth, or other sharp objects.
- Put the condom on after the penis is erect and before any genital, oral, or anal contact with the partner.
- Use only water-based lubricants (e.g., K-Y Jelly™, Astroglide™, AquaLube™, and glycerin) with latex condoms. Oil-based lubricants (e.g., petroleum jelly, shortening, mineral oil, massage oils, body lotions, and cooking oil) can weaken latex.
- Ensure adequate lubrication during vaginal and anal sex, which might require the use of exogenous water-based lubricants.
- To prevent the condom from slipping off, hold the condom firmly against the base of the penis during withdrawal, and withdraw while the penis is still erect.

Selected Resources

American Social Health Association (ASHA)
P.O. Box 13827
Research Triangle Park, NC 27709
919-361-8400
www.ashastd.org

Association of Reproductive Health Professionals
1901 L Street, NW, Suite 300
Washington, DC 20036
202-466-3825
www.arhp.org/

Centers for Disease Control and Prevention
National Center for HIV/AIDS, Viral
Hepatitis, STD, and TB Prevention
1600 Clifton Road
Atlanta, GA 30333
800-232-4636
www.cdc.gov/nchhstp/

World Health Organization
Avenue Appia 20
1211 Geneva 27
Switzerland
Phone: + 41 22 791 21 11
www.who.int/en/

References

Adler, M. W. (1980). The terrible peril: A historical perspective on the venereal diseases. *British Medical Journal, 281*(6234), 206-211.

American Social Health Association. (2010a). Herpes resource center: Learn about herpes - Fast facts. Retrieved December 8, 2010, from http://www.ashastd.org/herpes /herpes_learn.cfm

American Social Health Association. (2010b). HPV and Cervical Cancer Prevention Resource Center: Learn about HPV - Overview. Retrieved December 10, 2010, from http://www. ashastd.org/hpv/hpv_learn.cfm

American Social Health Association. (2010c). Learn about STIs/ STDs: Hepatitis - Fast facts. Retrieved December 13, 2010, from http://www.ashastd.org/learn/learn_hepatitis.cfm

American Social Health Association. (2010d). Learn about STIs/ STDs: HIV and AIDS - Overview. Retrieved December 10, 2010, from http://www.ashastd.org/learn /learn_hiv_aids_ overview.cfm

American Social Health Association. (2010e). Learn about STIs/ STDs: HIV and AIDS - Questions & answers - Risk reduction. Retrieved December 8, 2010, from http://www.ashastd.org/ learn/learn_hiv_aids_risk.cfm#q1

American Social Health Association. (2010f). Learn about STIs/ STDs: HIV and AIDS - Questions & answers - Testing. Retrieved December 8, 2010, from http://www.ashastd.org/ learn/learn_hiv_aids_testing.cfm

American Social Health Association. (2010g). Learn about STIs/ STDs: Overview. Retrieved December 8, 2010, from http:// www.ashastd.org/learn/learn_overview.cfm

American Social Health Association. (2010h). Sexual health: Talking to your child about sex and sexual health. Retrieved December 13, 2010, from http://www.ashastd.org/ sexualhealth/talking. cfm

American Social Health Association. (2010i). Sexual health: What is sexual health? Retrieved December 13, 2010, from http://www. ashastd.org/sexualhealth/index.cfm

Centers for Disease Control and Prevention. (2007). Sexually transmitted diseases (STDs): Trichomoniasis - CDC fact sheet. Retrieved December 13, 2010, from http://www.cdc.gov/std/ trichomonas/STDFact-Trichomoniasis.htm

Centers for Disease Control and Prevention. (2009). Sexually transmitted diseases (STDs): Genital HPV infection - Fact sheet. Retrieved December 10, 2010, from http://www.cdc.gov/ std/HPV/STDFact-HPV.htm

Centers for Disease Control and Prevention. (2010a). *Sexually transmitted disease surveillance 2009.* Atlanta, GA: U.S. Department of Health and Human Services.

Centers for Disease Control and Prevention. (2010b). Sexually transmitted diseases (STDs): Chlamydia - CDC fact sheet. Retrieved December 8, 2010, from http://www.cdc.gov/std/ chlamydia/STDFact-Chlamydia.htm

Centers for Disease Control and Prevention. (2010c). Sexually transmitted diseases (STDs): Genital herpes - CDC fact sheet. Retrieved December 9, 2010, from http://www.cdc.gov/std/ Herpes/STDFact-Herpes.htm

Centers for Disease Control and Prevention. (2010d). Sexually transmitted diseases (STDs): Gonorrhea - CDC fact sheet. Retrieved December 9, 2010, from http://www.cdc.gov/std/gonorrhea/STDFact-gonorrhea.htm

Centers for Disease Control and Prevention. (2010e). Viral Hepatitis scientific information - Populations at risk: STDs and viral Hepatitis. Retrieved December 13, 2010, from http://www.cdc.gov/hepatitis/Populations/STDs.htm

Centers for Disease Control and Prevention. (2011). Sexually transmitted diseases. Retrieved April 26, 2011, from http://www.cdc.gov/std/

Fleming, D. T., & Wasserheit, J. N. (1999). From epidemiological synergy to public health policy and practice: The contribution of other sexually transmitted diseases to sexual transmission of HIV infection. *Sexually Transmitted Infections, 75*, 3-17.

Mayo Clinic staff. (2010). HIV/AIDS: Causes. Retrieved April 26, 2011, from http://www.mayoclinic.com/health/hiv-aids/DS00005/DSECTION=causes

Pan American Health Organization & World Health Organization. (2000). *Promotion of sexual health: Recommendations for action.* Proceedings of a Regional Consultation, Antigua Guatemala, Guatemala. Retrieved April 26, 2011, from http://www.paho.org/English/AD /FCH /AI/PromotionSexualHealth.pdf

Sacco, L. (2004). Venereal disease. In *Encyclopedia of children and childhood in history and society.* Retrieved April 26, 2011, from http://www.encyclopedia.com/topic /venereal_disease.aspx

Workowski, K. A., & Berman, S. M. (2006). Sexually transmitted diseases treatment guidelines, 2006. *Morbidity and Mortality Weekly Report, 55*(RR-11), 1-94.

DRUG ABUSE AND ADDICTION

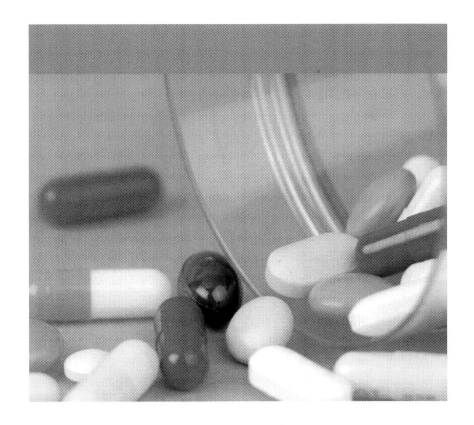

D rug abuse, or substance abuse, severely threatens U.S. public health. Drug abuse is the use of drugs in a manner or amount inconsistent with the medical or social patterns of a culture (Hanson, 2010), and it costs Americans 100,000 lives annually (National Institute on Drug Abuse [NIDA], 2008). Commonly abused drugs in the US are alcohol, tobacco, prescription drugs, heroin, inhalants, marijuana, and cocaine. Abuse of these and other drugs can change both the structure of the brain and how the brain functions. Individuals use drugs for a variety of reasons, but scientists believe that these changes in the brain explain users' destructive behaviors and continued drug use. Drug abuse is associated with spousal and child abuse, motor-vehicle-related death, injury, sexually transmitted disease, unintended pregnancy, school failure, increased health-care cost, and lower worker productivity (U.S. Department of Health and Human Services [HHS], 2000).

Substance abuse can lead to addiction. Addiction is a chronic, relapsing brain disease characterized by compulsive drug seeking and use, despite harmful consequences (NIDA, 2008). According to NIDA (n.d.a), drug addiction is a treatable type of brain disease. Substance abuse can also lead to dependence upon the substance to avoid withdrawal or in order to feel the ability to function normally in society.

The abuse of alcohol and other drugs negatively impacts one's quality of life. Babies born to drug-abusing mothers suffer from increased risk of physical, mental, and emotional consequences. Drug-abusing adolescents suffer academic failures, unplanned pregnancies, violence, and medical consequences. Adults abusing drugs have difficulty with attention, learning, memory, and negative relationship and work consequences (NIDA, 2008). The medical consequences of drug abuse and addiction include heart disease, cancer, stroke, HIV/AIDS, hepatitis B and C, lung disease, obesity, and mental disorders (NIDA, 2008). This abuse can also bring about chronic diseases, such as liver disease and premature death. Alcohol and tobacco use in particular have been cited among the top causes of preventable death in the United States (Mokdad, Marks, Stroup, & Gerberding, 2004).

Sociocultural Influences

The history of addiction in America dates back to the 1700s when Native American tribes attempted to decrease the use of alcohol among their people. The first American essay on alcoholism was written in 1774, depicting alcohol as a destroyer of human life (National Council on Alcoholism and Drug Dependence [NCADD], n.d.). Drugs like alcohol, cannabis, and heroin were used in products advertised to fight general aches and pains. These products were available to the general public during the 1800s as there were no laws or regulations by any government entity until the early 1900s (Hanson, 2010). Individuals would take these products and become addicted without fully understanding the dangers of using them. Laws continued to be passed and enforced during the early 1900s in order to decrease drug abuse and addiction. There was a resurgence of attention on drug abuse and addiction during the 1960s when drugs like psychedelics, marijuana, and amphetamines gained in popularity within public view. The Drug Enforcement Administration (DEA) was created in 1973 to assist with attempts to control the distribution and use of drugs (NCADD, n.d.). Despite new laws and enforcement, drug use continued in the US and hit its highest mark up to that date in 1979 when 1 in 10 Americans reported using drugs regularly. Drugs continued to be popular as the price and availability of drugs became less of a barrier to more Americans throughout the 1980s. During the 1990s until now, drugs continue to be available and accessible as do the dangers associated with abuse of the substances ("Illegal Drugs," n.d.). Many programs for drug-use prevention and addiction exist throughout the US. Science has come a long way in helping to understand the process of addiction and the health consequences that come from both short- and long-term drug abuse.

Biologically, certain genes can influence an individual's risk factors for developing abuse or addiction tendencies. Individuals whose parent or parents suffer from addiction are at a higher risk of suffering from addiction. Drug addiction also often occurs along with mental illness. Mental illness can precede addiction or can be brought about by drug abuse in those who have vulnerabilities, such as chemical imbalances (NIDA, 2008).

Environmental influences that can increase one's chances of abuse or addiction are witnessing violence, stress, drug availability, and early physical or sexual abuse (NIDA, 2008). Peer drug use can also increase the risk for drug abuse and addiction, especially during adolescence (NIDA, 2003). Age at first use of alcohol or other drugs is another factor associated with abuse or addiction. The younger one starts using alcohol or drugs, the more likely they will abuse drugs later in life or suffer from addiction (Substance Abuse and Mental Health Services Administration [SAMHSA], Office of Applied Studies, 2008).

Alcohol and drug abuse often co-occur causing users to suffer from more severe dependence issues as well as psychiatric disorders. In addition to suffering health consequences, such as liver and heart disease, these users are more likely to attempt suicide (Arnaout & Petrakis, 2008).

Alcohol

A standard drink of alcohol is any drink that contains about 14 g (about 0.6 fluid oz or 1.2 tablespoons) of pure alcohol. This is the amount of alcohol usually found in one 12-oz beer, one 4- to 5-oz glass of wine, or one 1.5-oz shot of 80-proof liquor (NIDA, n.d.a). Heavy drinking is defined as having 4 or more drinks on the same occasion for women and 5 or more drinks on the same occasion for men 5 nights or more in a 30-day period (SAMHSA, 2009b). The *Dietary Guidelines for Americans* from the U.S. Department of Agriculture (USDA) recommends that daily intake of alcohol be limited to 1 drink per day for women and 2 drinks per day for men (HSS & USDA, 2008). In addition, the USDA recommends that the following list of individuals refrain from drinking alcohol all together:

- Children and adolescents.
- Individuals of any age who cannot limit their drinking to low levels.
- Women who may become pregnant or who are pregnant.
- Individuals who plan to drive, operate machinery, or take part in other activities that require attention, skill, or coordination.
- Individuals taking prescription or over-the-counter medications that can interact with alcohol.
- Individuals with certain medical conditions.
- Persons recovering from alcoholism.

In the 2008 National Health Interview Survey, 51% of U.S. adults reported regular drinking (12 drinks in the past year), while 14% reported 1-11 drinks in the last year (SAMHSA, 2009b). The National Survey on Drug Use and Health (NSDUH) conducted by the Substance Abuse and Mental Health Services Association also looks at annual drug use among Americans. This survey asks participants about drug use in the month prior to the study, use during the year preceding the study, and lifetime use. The 2008 NSDUH indicated that past-month alcohol use among 12-17 year olds declined steadily from 17.6% in 2002 to 15.9% in 2007. It decreased to 14.6% in 2008 (SAMHSA, 2009b). Heavy drinking numbers have stayed consistent at approximately 17.3 million people from 2007 to 2008. Up to 70% of adolescents 19-20 years of age are categorized as heavy drinkers (SAMHSA, 2009b).

The 2008 NSDUH also indicated over one quarter (28.1%) of persons aged 12-20 (an estimated 10.8 million persons) used alcohol in the past month. More than half (51.1%) of those aged 18-20 were current alcohol users compared with 25.9% of those aged 15-17 and 6.1% of those aged 12-14. Underage males were more likely than their female counterparts to be current alcohol users (28.8% vs. 27.4%).

Specific Effects on the Young

Drinking alcohol can negatively affect the brain development and functioning of young people under the age of 15 years. Youth who drink before age 15 are more likely to have other substance abuse problems when compared to peers who do not. Those who begin drinking before 15 years of age are also more likely to report risky sexual behaviors, be involved in car crashes, suffer unintentional injuries, and participate in physical fights through adolescence and on into adulthood (HHS, 2007).

General Effects on Health

Drinking alcohol in amounts greater than recommended by the USDA can result in health complications, such as cancer, heart disease, and unintentional injuries or death (National Institute on Alcohol Abuse and Alcoholism [NIAAA], 1993). According to the American Cancer Society (2007), the more a person drinks, the more the risk for developing cancer. The American Heart Association (2010) links increased alcohol intake with higher levels of triglycerides in the blood, increased blood pressure, increased incidence of heart failure, and increased caloric intake.

The increased triglyceride levels associated with moderate to high levels of alcohol use are also connected to an increased risk of cardiovascular disease (Ghandi & Raina, 1984). High blood cholesterol and triglyceride levels are known to increase risk for heart disease. Triglycerides are the main energy source in blood. Levels exceeding the recommended ratio of triglycerides serve to increase inflammation of the pancreas and encourage atherosclerosis ("High Cholesterol," n.d.).

Moderate to high levels of alcohol consumption increase blood pressure in both men and women, the more one drinks causing the greatest increases (Malinski, Sesso, Lopez-Jimenez, Buring,

& Gaziano, 2004; Thadhani et al., 2002). Untreated chronic high blood pressure damages the heart and its blood vessels, leading to increased risk of heart disease, including heart failure. Heart failure occurs when the muscle of the heart can no longer pump blood effectively. This condition occurs over time and is most often caused by high blood pressure, coronary artery disease, or diabetes. Heart failure is a chronic medical condition that requires medical follow-up on a regular basis. Approximately 5 million people in the US have heart failure and about 300,000 die annually from it (National Heart, Blood, & Lung Institute, 2010).

Alcohol ingestion affects the entire brain and central nervous system as well. People who drink 14 or more drinks per week on a regular basis experience brain shrinkage, the greatest effect among women over 70 years of age (Reinberg, 2007). Heavy alcohol use causes damage to the brain, liver, and heart of women at a much faster rate than to men (Leigh, 2007). In the United States, alcohol abuse and hepatitis C are the leading causes of cirrhosis of the liver, and cirrhosis of the liver is the cause of over 80% of U.S. liver cancer cases (American Liver Foundation, 2010). Cirrhosis of the liver causes over 27,000 deaths in the US annually.

Health Benefits From Alcohol Consumption

Drinking alcohol in the recommended amounts can actually work to decrease risk for cardiovascular disease (Mayo Clinic staff, 2011). Moderate alcohol consumption has also been shown to provide other health benefits, such as lowered risk of type 2 diabetes, gallstones, stroke (especially transient ischemic attacks), peripheral artery disease, and decreased risk of death from a heart attack (Koppes, Dekker, Hendriks, Bouter, & Heine, 2005; Mukamal, Maclure, Muller, Sherwood, & Mittleman, 2001; Muntwyler, Hennekens, Buring, & Gaziano, 1998; Solomon et al., 2000). The key to receiving the benefits from alcohol consumption is for a person to drink the daily recommended amounts (1 drink for women per day; 2 drinks for men per day).

Binge Drinking

Public health officials are very concerned about binge drinking. Binge drinking is having 5 or more drinks for males or 4 or more drinks for females in a single occasion (NIAAA, 2004). Binge drinking is most common among the late-teen to early-twenties age group (Naimi, Brewer, Mokdad, Denny, & Serdula, 2003; SAMHSA, 2004.). Data from 2008 indicate that 58.1 million people 12 and older participate in binge drinking. This translates to 1 out of every 5 people 12 and older binge drinking (SAMHSA, 2009b). Teens drink less frequently than adults, but when they drink, they drink larger quantities (HHS, 2007). Estimates from the 2006 NSDUH (SAMHSA, 2007) indicated there were 11 million underage drinkers in the United States. In addition, 7.2 million youth ages 12-20 years were considered binge drinkers. Binge drinking rates among the 18-25 age group from the 2008 NSDUH were at 41%, while the heavy drinking rate was 14.5%, both similar to 2007 results (SAMHSA, 2009b).

According to the Higher Education Center for Alcohol, Drug Abuse, and Violence Prevention, binge and heavy drinking are among the most widespread health problems at U.S. colleges and universities. Approximately 80% of college students drink alcohol with a national average for binge drinking at about 40%, and 20% report heavy episodic drinking, which is defined as 3 or more binge drinking episodes within 2 weeks. Alcohol consumption is associated with academic consequences, illicit drug use, and tobacco use (HHS, 2007).

Binge drinking also causes alcohol poisoning. Alcohol poisoning can cause a coma and is a serious and potentially lethal consequence of drinking large quantities of alcohol. Binge drinking increases blood alcohol concentration (BAC) to a dangerous level in a short time period. At a high enough BAC, alcohol can depress the functioning of the central nervous system. Individuals' gag reflexes, heart rates, and breathing would be affected. If enough alcohol has been consumed, they may pass out. Even when passed out, their BAC may still continue to rise, placing them at a greater risk of dying from alcohol poisoning. If untreated, victims may vomit and choke. They may also suffer from hypothermia or hypoglycemia (which can lead to seizures), and the dehydration from vomiting can cause seizures, brain damage, or death. Respirations that drop below 8 breaths per minute put the individual at risk of respiratory or cardiac emergencies as well. Even if victims survive, they may suffer irreversible brain damage (NIAAA, n.d.).

Unintentional Injuries and Alcohol

Drinking alcohol in irresponsible ways, such as drinking and driving, underage drinking, and binge drinking, leads to unintentional injuries and death worldwide. The World Health Organization (WHO, 2007) reports that 10%-18% of global emergency room injury visits are related to alcohol consumption. Costs associated with impaired driving that causes unintentional injury in the United States top more than $51 billion on an annual basis (Blincoe et al., 2002). According to the CDC (2008), excessive alcohol use, including heavy drinking and binge drinking, is the third leading cause of lifestyle-related death in the US.

Individuals who drink heavy amounts of alcohol are more likely to become violent than those who do not. Alcohol-induced aggression is a factor in intentional and unintentional injuries associated with alcohol consumption (Arseneault, Moffitt, Caspi, Taylor, & Silva, 2000; Collins & Messerschmidt, 1993; Cunradi, Caetano, Clark, & Schafer, 1999; Higley, n.d.; Scott, Schafer, & Greenfield, 1999). Alcohol use is also linked to unwanted sexual behaviors, including acquaintance rape, unplanned pregnancy, and high-risk sexual behaviors (CDC, Office of Women's Health, 2009; Corbin, Bernat, Calhoun, McNair, & Seals, 2001). Adolescents who drink alcohol are more likely to engage in risky sexual behaviors, such as unprotected sex (Leigh & Stall, 1993).

According to the National Institute of Justice, alcohol use leads to increased aggressiveness and altered interpretations of sexual interest among college-aged students. Approximately 50% of sexual assaults are associated with alcohol consumption on behalf of both the victim and perpetrator (Abbey, McAuslan, & Ross, 1998;

Abbey, Ross, McDuffie, & McAuslan, 1996). Other risk factors for female victims of sexual assault include drug use, attending a college or university with a high drinking rate, belonging to a sorority, and drinking heavily during their high school years (CDC, Office of Women's Health, 2009). A 2008 study by New York City's Department of Health states that people who binge drink report more sexual partners than those who refrain from binge drinking, and the higher the number of sexual partners, the higher the rate of sexually transmitted infections and unplanned pregnancies (New York City Department of Health and Mental Hygiene, 2009).

Pregnant women who drink alcohol are at risk for injuring their unborn child. Alcohol use during pregnancy can cause fetal alcohol syndrome in the developing fetus. Fetal alcohol syndrome, the leading cause of mental retardation, is 100% preventable if pregnant women do not drink (CDC, 2009). Fetal alcohol syndrome is associated with facial abnormalities, growth retardation, and brain damage usually displayed as intellectual and behavioral difficulties (NIAAA, 2000).

Unintentional Death and Alcohol

Injuries are the leading cause of death for individuals 21 years of age and under. Alcohol is a leading contributor to this trend. Alcohol-related injuries are responsible for about 5,000 deaths annually in the 21-and-under age group. Of these 5,000 deaths, 38% are from motor vehicle crashes, 32% from homicides, and 6% from suicides (HHS, 2007).

Data from the 2007 National Highway Traffic Safety Administration (NHTSA, 2009) Traffic Safety Facts indicated that alcohol-impaired-driving fatalities accounted for 32% of all motor vehicle fatalities in the US. Impaired driving is when the driver has a blood alcohol concentration (BAC) of .08 or greater. In 2010, there were 10,228 fatalities where BAC was .08 or greater. (Traffic Safety Facts, 2012). From 12 midnight to 3 a.m., the number of all traffic fatalities associated with alcohol-impaired driving jumped to 64%

According to the NHTSA, 3 out of 10 Americans will be involved in an alcohol-related traffic crash during their lifetime

(NHTSA, 2001). Alcohol-related fatalities occur when either the driver or non-occupant involved in the crash has a BAC of .01 or higher. In 2007, 31% of fatalities of youth 15-20 years of age involved drivers with BACs of .01 or greater, while 26% had BACs of .08 or greater (NHTSA, 2009).

Although alcohol-impaired-driving fatalities are greater than 30% of all annual fatalities, the numbers have been decreasing over the years. A NHTSA study examined impaired driving throughout the US in 1973, 1986, 1996, and 2007. Results from this study showed a 71% decline in alcohol-impaired driving during weekend nighttime hours (Compton & Berning, 2009). Drinking and driving has decreased from 2002 to 2008 by about 2%, from 14.2% to 12.4%, with the highest rate of drinking and driving between the ages of 21 to 26 years old (SAMHSA, 2009b). Efforts to decrease the rate of drinking and driving are needed to further decrease the rate of associated fatalities in the US.

Marijuana

Marijuana is the most commonly abused illicit substance in the United States. According to the National Institute on Drug Abuse (NIDA, 2004), more than 94 million Americans 12 and older have tried marijuana at least once in their lifetime. Nora Volkow, Director of NIDA, states that marijuana can produce negative side effects in its users, including addiction (NIDA, 2011). Marijuana use can harm the lungs in a way similar to tobacco (Sarafian, Magallanes, Shau, Tashkin, & Roth, 1999). In addition, marijuana use can lead to impaired brain development in youth (Brook, Rosen, & Brook, 2001). Other consequences include impaired short-term memory as well as impaired verbal skills and judgment (Volkow, 2005). The negative impact on one's memory increases with the more one uses the drug. Research among college students showed that students who smoked marijuana 27 out of 30 days had significant declines in attention, memory, and learning skills after 24 hours of drug abstinence when compared to students who smoked 3 out of 30 days (Pope & Yurgelun-Todd, 1996). Marijuana use has also been shown to cause deterioration in emotional and problem-solving skills (Scheier & Botvin, 1996). Motor coordination, sensory perception, reaction time, and glare recovery are also impaired with the use of marijuana (Hanson, 2009); therefore, one should not drive a car or operate heavy machinery while under the influence of marijuana.

According to the National Survey on Drug Use and Health, adults reporting marijuana use in the last month held steady at 8% for 2007 and 2008 (SAMHSA, 2009a). Marijuana use within the last month among high school seniors showed a slight increase, from 18.8% in 2007 to 19.4% in 2008, and 10th graders showed a modest decline in last-month marijuana use at 14.2% in 2007 and 13.8% in 2008 (SAMHSA, 2008). Among the 12-17 age group, marijuana use in the last month declined from 8.2% in 2002 to 6.8% in 2005 and has stayed steady at 6.7% since. In 2002, 32.4% of youth 12-17 perceived a great level of risk associated with one-time marijuana use in the last month. In 2007, 34.5% of youth 12-17 perceived a great level of risk associated with marijuana use in the last month. When youth perceive a great level of risk associated with using a drug, their reported use of the substance is lower than when they perceive a low level of risk from using a substance (SAMHSA, 2009a).

Prescription Drugs

Prescription drug abusers use prescription drugs in excess or for reasons other than prescribed, or they take medication that has not been prescribed to them. This abuse can cause serious health implications. Depending on the drug and amount taken, abusing these substances can cause heart rhythm irregularities, seizures, dangerously high body temperatures, anxiety, and even paranoia (NIDA, n.d.b). According to NIDA, as of 2009, prescription drugs are the second most commonly abused substance after marijuana in the US (Volkow, 2011). Like other drug abuse, prescription drug abuse can change the way the brain functions and lead to addiction.

Opioids or opiates, otherwise known as narcotics, are often

prescribed because of their effective pain-management qualities. They are frequently abused. Common opioids are morphine, codeine, and oxycodone. Individuals who stop using opioids or decrease the dosage can experience withdrawal symptoms. These symptoms can be uncomfortable and include diarrhea, goose bumps, restlessness, insomnia, muscle and bone pain, vomiting, and involuntary leg movements. Large doses or a single large dose of this category of drug can severely depress one's respiratory system, causing a life-threatening situation.

Central nervous system depressants are another commonly abused prescription substance among Americans. This category, which includes benzodiazepines and barbiturates, is often used to treat anxiety and sleep disorders because these drugs slow brain function. Central nervous system depressants cause users to build a tolerance to the drug's effects; therefore, users are inclined to increase doses of the drug to continue to feel its effects. Long-term use of the drug can lead to physical dependence. When users stop using it or reduce the dose, they will suffer withdrawal, which can cause the brain to race out of control, leading to seizures or other harmful health consequences. Withdrawal from prolonged use of most depressants can have life-threatening consequences, but withdrawal from benzodiazepines can just be uncomfortable and problemsome and is usually not life-threatening (NIDA, n.d.b).

Club drugs like GHB and Rohypnol are also central nervous system depressants and can also produce negative consequences when abused. Used in date-rape situations, the drugs can cause a person to become amnesiac and incapacitated quickly. Coma, seizures, respiratory difficulties, and even death can occur from the misuse of these drugs or by combining them with other drugs such as alcohol (NIDA, 2010c).

Another category of abused prescription drugs is central nervous system stimulants. These drugs cause an increase in energy, alertness, and attention. With brand names such as Ritalin, Adderall, and Concerta, stimulants are commonly prescribed to treat narcolepsy and attention deficit and hyperactivity disorders. When these drugs are prescribed by a physician, the dose is slowly increased until a therapeutic level is reached. The problem with abuse of these drugs is that users will quickly increase doses or administer the drug in ways that interrupt the brain's normal communication process between cells. Abuse of these drugs leads to increased dosing, which can cause irregular heartbeat, cardiovascular failure, seizures, or dangerously high body temperature in the user. For a user who combines stimulants and other drugs, such as antidepressants or decongestants, danger occurs in the form of high blood pressure and heartbeat irregularities (NIDA, 2009).

Cocaine and Heroin

Cocaine is a central nervous system stimulant that is smoked, snorted, or injected. It can also be processed into rock crystals to form crack cocaine. Cocaine causes an increase in heart rate, body temperature, and blood pressure. It is hard on the cardiovascular system and can cause heart attack, stroke, respiratory failure, seizures, abdominal pain, and nausea, even upon first-time use. It is most frequently abused along with alcohol, which is the most common drug combination that results in death (NIDA, 2010a).

In 2008, reported cocaine use by Americans 12 years and older was 5.3 million, and crack use within the last year of the study was reported by 1.1 million Americans (SAMHSA, 2009b). Approximately 7% of Americans reported having tried cocaine at least once by their senior year in high school. Current reports indicate 1 in 6 Americans having tried cocaine by their 30th birthday (NIDA, 2010a).

Heroin is a highly addictive, illegal opiate. The heroin found on the streets is often cut or bulked up with toxic substances, leaving users at risk of not knowing its true contents. Heroin can be injected, snorted, or smoked and can cause death, overdose, or transmission of HIV and other blood-borne pathogens via needle sharing. Physiological effects from heroin include slowing of the cardiovascular and respiratory systems, which can be fatal. Negative medical consequences include collapsed veins, lung complications, bacterial infections of blood vessels and heart valves, abscesses, and kidney and liver disease. Because heroin crosses the blood-brain barrier and quickly enters the brain, addiction occurs quickly. In 2003, 3.7 million Americans reported heroin use at some point during their lifetime while 119,000 reported use within the last month of the survey being conducted. Of those who reported past-year use, 57.4% were classified as dependent upon heroin or heroin abusers, while 281,000 received treatment for heroin abuse (NIDA, 2005).

Inhalants

Inhalants are chemicals frequently found around the home that contain vapors the user inhales to get a quick high. Common household products, such as gasoline, paint thinners, glues, whip cream canisters, hair spray, spray paints, and cleaning fluids, are used as inhalants. The short-term effects of the intoxicants are a high similar to moderate alcohol use; however, inhaling large amounts can produce a toxic effect, causing loss of sensation and even loss of consciousness. Health consequences associated with inhalant use and abuse include negative effects on the kidneys, liver, heart, and brain as well as irreparable neurotoxin effects to the nervous system and brain.

In addition, users may experience rapid heart rhythms and sudden sniffing death syndrome, a condition where the user's heart fails to continue functioning causing death. Death by abuse of inhalants can also occur through asphyxiation, suffocation, seizures, coma, choking, or participating in a behavior that causes a fatal injury (NIDA, 2010b). Inhalants are a category of drugs where abuse is concentrated mostly among the younger population. NIDA's Monitoring the Future study states that 15.7% of eighth graders have used inhalants. According to the 2008 NSDUH, 729,000 people 12 and older reported trying an inhalant in the past year, and 70% of them were 18 and under. The short- and long-term health implications for abuse of inhalants are serious and must be addressed in order to decrease abuse of these substances.

An interview on personal experience with alcohol and drugs was conducted with Laura, a 55-year-old woman. Laura's story begins with growing up in a house with a built-in bar, which made her think every house had one. Before school, she would drink from the keg on her patio. Her parents drank every night and smoked as long as she could remember. Laura began smoking marijuana in high school, and then after marrying her first husband, she experimented with other drugs.

Addiction took over Laura's life. During that time, she did not think much of herself and did not possess the courage to confront her past. She let her addiction dictate her actions, telling her what to do and how to do it. Because of it, she almost lost her family and her house. Laura has also suffered from several health issues due to her drug use. She continues to endure memory loss from a brain aneurysm that resulted from her addiction.

Laura's path to recovery began when she became dedicated to ending that madness in her life. Realizing that she was a worthy person, Laura found herself, her truth, and the courage to address the issues of her past. From her own experience, Laura recommends the encouragement of a 12-step recovery program and the recognition that God created us and that we are all worthwhile.

For a personal account of how tobacco, alcohol, and drugs affected one's health, we interviewed Jacob, a 63-year-old male. As a teen, Jacob smoked cigarettes and drank. He became an alcoholic when he joined the military and stayed overseas. After Jacob came home, he experimented with methamphetamine and used IV drugs for 16 years. At its worst, his meth addiction cost him $400 per week. He had also dealt drugs while his alcoholism and meth use continued.

Keeping a job during this time became difficult for Jacob. His meth use and sleep deprivation caused him to be late for work and job interviews. He also missed the social gatherings that he was invited to. Jacob remained a smoker during this time even though he had asthma, leading him to suffer border-line emphysema. He also became angry and aggressive and began to lie, cheat, and steal.

Jacob isolated himself and lost several jobs. He lost his home and alienated his family, including his children.

When Jacob was an addict, he felt he was insane. He made bad decisions and his relationships fell apart. He and his wife had been using drugs together, and she called him a "junkie." Her hypocrisy and being called a "junkie" infuriated Jacob to the point of quitting his drug use for the next 10 years. That was only the beginning to his recovery. After Jacob quit, he was extremely judgmental and teeming with rage and verbal abuse. Only enrollment in a 12-step program and a sponsor provided what he needed to move toward a successful recovery.

From there, Jacob started to regain feelings and emotions that had lain dormant for years, which he found difficult to process. Regular meetings and his sponsor helped him through this welcome difficulty. Their guidance made Jacob concentrate on his sobriety, altering his perspective on life. All of this lead him back to the family and children he had mistreated due to his drug use.

Jacob had needed to want to recover from his addictions and ask for help to facilitate his success. For him, help came in various forms, such as a certain speaker at a meeting, a simple encouraging word, a concerned friend, and even an angry response to his behavior. Today, Jacob sponsors other men and conducts 12-step programs. He tells recovering addicts that, first, they must decide to quit drugs and alcohol and truly desire to quit: Without that, they will fail because only that will enable them to take the various paths to recovery, such as detox, drug and alcohol programs, AA or NA meetings, or a 12-step program. Jacob follows Terence Gorski's seven governing principles of recovery and relapse prevention. He has learned from Gorski that addiction is a process and that the triggers of relapse must be known because relapse is also a process.

Jacob now looks to Jesus Christ and centers on Him instead of drugs and alcohol. He has refocused his attention away from his addictions. That necessary action has strengthened him. Jacob has not used meth for over 23 years and has not had a drink for the past 10. He thinks his success over addiction is based on a certain sanity and the constructive changes that impact lives, his and others. To him, failure is insanity, doing the same thing time and time again, thinking that each time will end differently.

Conclusion

Drug abuse and addiction directly impact users *and* those around them in a negative way via medical, social, economic, and criminal justice consequences. Costs associated with drug abuse and addiction top $484 billion annually. That includes medical expenditures, crime, accidents, lost productivity, and earnings. Environmental and biological factors can play a role in the development of addiction and drug abuse. Progress is being made in the decrease of alcohol addiction, but the alcohol abuse rate is still increasing. Drinking by college students accounts for approximately 1,700 deaths, 600,000 injuries, 700,000 assaults, and more than 97,000 sexual assaults annually (Hingson, Ralph, et al.).

The health consequences for abuse of all illicit drugs and prescription drugs have serious costs to society. Prevention efforts made by professionals who study drug abuse and prevention and NIDA have doubled in both size and scope since their preventive efforts began in 1997 with the introduction of *Preventing Drug Use Among Children and Adolescents: A Research-Based Guide for Parents, Educators, and Community Leaders* (NIDA, 2003). In the US, efforts to continue research in drug abuse prevention must continue, while efforts to treat drug addiction must increase in order to cut costs associated with both issues.

Recommendations

In order to decrease drug abuse and addiction in the US, a concerted effort between law enforcement, policy makers, communities, families, and health and social service agencies is needed (U.S. Department of Justice, 2000). Families, schools, and communities serve a vital role in recognizing risk factors and providing protective factors to those at risk for drug abuse or addiction problems. Risk factors increase the chance that a person will abuse drugs while protective factors serve to protect a person from abuse of drugs (NIDA, 2003). Efforts to decrease risk factors and increase protective factors include the use of prevention programs at community levels. NIDA recommends 16 prevention principles for communities and families in the effort to reduce the abuse of drugs. Each principal contains steps to address interventions or prevention through planning, implementation, and evaluation (NIDA, 2003, pp. 2-5).

Selected Resources

Community Anti-Drug Coalitions of America (CADCA)
901 North Pitt Street, Suite 300
Alexandria, VA 22314
800-542-2322
www.cadca.org

Drug Strategies, Inc.
1150 Connecticut Avenue, NW, Suite 800
Washington, DC 20036
202-289-9070
www.drugstrategies.org

National Institute on Alcohol Abuse and Alcoholism (NIAAA)
5635 Fishers Lane, MSC 9304
Bethesda, MD 20892
301-443-3860
www.niaaa.nih.gov

National Institute on Drug Abuse (NIDA)
9000 Rockville Pike
Bethesda, MD 20892
301-443-1124
www.nida.nih.gov

References

Abbey, A., McAuslan, P., & Ross, L. T. (1998). Sexual assault perpetration by college men: The role of alcohol, misperception of sexual intent, and sexual beliefs and experiences. *Journal of Social and Clinical Psychology, 17,* 167-195.

Abbey, A., Ross, L. T., McDuffie, D., & McAuslan, P. (1996). Alcohol and dating risk factors for sexual assault among college women. *Psychology of Women Quarterly, 20,* 147-169.

American Cancer Society. (2007). *Alcohol and cancer.* Retrieved from http://www.cancer.org/acs/groups/content/@ healthpromotions/documents/document/acsq-017622.pdf

American Liver Foundation. (2010). Alcohol-related liver disease. Retrieved January 5, 2010, from http://www.liverfoundation. org/abouttheliver/info/alcohol/

American Heart Association. (2010). Alcohol, wine, and cardiovascular disease. Retrieved January 5, 2010, from http:// www.americanheart.org /presenter.jhtml?identifier=4422

Arnaout, B., & Petrakis, I. (2008). Diagnosing co-morbid drug use in patients with alcohol use disorders. *Alcohol Research & Health, 31*(2), 148-154.

Arseneault, L., Moffitt, T. E., Caspi, A., Taylor, P. J., & Silva, P. A. (2000). Mental disorders and violence in a total birth cohort: Results from the Dunedin study. *Archives of General Psychiatry, 57,* 979-986.

Blincoe, L., Seay, A., Zaloshnja, E., Miller, T., Romano, E., Luchter, S., & Spicer R. (2002). *The economic impact of motor vehicle crashes, 2000* (Report No. DOT HS 809 446). Retrieved from National Highway Traffic Safety Administration website: http://www.nhtsa.gov/DOT/NHTSA/Communication%20 &%20Consumer%20Information/Articles/Associated%20 Files/EconomicImpact2000.pdf

Brook, J. S., Rosen, Z., & Brook, D. W. (2001). The effect of early marijuana use on later anxiety and depressive symptoms. *NYS Psychologist,* 35-39.

Centers for Disease Control and Prevention. (2009). Fetal alcohol spectrum disorders (FASDs): Facts about FASDs. Retrieved January 5, 2009, from http://cdc.gov/ncbddd/fasd/index.html

Centers for Disease Control and Prevention, Office of Women's Health. (2009). Family health: College health and safety. Retrieved February 5, 2010, from http://www.cdc.gov/family/ college/

Collins, J. J., & Messerschmidt, M. A. (1993). Epidemiology of alcohol-related violence. *Alcohol Health & Research World, 17,* 93-100.

Compton, R., & Berning, A. (2009). *Traffic safety facts - Research note: Results of the 2007 National Roadside Survey of Alcohol and Drug Use by Drivers* (Publication No. DOT HS 811 175). Retrieved from http://www.nhtsa.gov/DOT/NHTSA/ Traffic%20Injury%20Control/Articles/Associated%20 Files/811175.pdf

Corbin, W., Bernat, J., Calhoun, K, McNair, L., & Seals, K. (2001). Role of alcohol expectancies and alcohol consumption among sexually victimized and nonvictimized college women. *Journal of Interpersonal Violence, 16,* 297-311.

Cunradi, C. B., Caetano, R., Clark, C. L., & Schafer, J. (1999). Alcohol-related problems and intimate partner violence among

White, Black, and Hispanic couples in the U.S. *Alcoholism: Clinical and Experimental Research, 23*, 1492-1501.

Gandhi, B. M., & Raina, N. (1984). Alcohol-induced changes in lipids and lipoproteins. *Alcoholism: Clinical and Experiential Research, 8*, 29-32.

Hanson, G.R. Venturelli, P.J., Fleckenstein, A.E. (2011). Drugs and Society, Eleventh Edition. Jones and Bartlett Learning: Boston, MA.

High cholesterol and triglyceride levels. (n.d.). Retrieved January 8, 2010, from Johns Hopkins Health Alerts website: http://www.johnshopkinshealthalerts.com/symptoms_remedies / hyperlipidemia/91-1.html

Higley, D. (n.d.). Individual differences in alcohol-induced aggression: A nonhuman-primate model. Retrieved from http://74.125.95.132/search?q=cache:ZVV0WyPIfkAJ:pubs. niaaa.nih.gov/publications/arh25-1/12-19.htm

Hingson, R. et al. Magnitude of Alcohol-Related Mortality and Morbidity Among U.S. College Students Ages 18-24: Changes from 1998 to 2001. Annual Review of Public Health, vol. 26, 259-79; 2005

Illegal drugs in America: *A modern history*. (n.d.). Retrieved May 26, 2011, from Drug Enforcement Administration Museum & Visitors Center website: http://www.deamuseum.org/museum_ ida.html

Koppes, L. L., Dekker, J. M., Hendriks, H. F., Bouter, L. M., & Heine, R. J. (2005). Moderate alcohol consumption lowers the risk of type 2 diabetes: A meta–analysis of prospective observational studies. Diabetes Care, *28*, 719-725.

Leigh, B., & Stall, R. (1993). Substance use and risky sexual behavior for exposure to HIV: Issues in methodology, interpretation, and prevention. *American Psychologist, 48,* 1035-1043.

Leigh, S. (2007, April 27). A woman's brain hit harder by alcohol abuse. *The Washington Post.* Retrieved from http://www. washingtonpost.com

Malinski, M. K., Sesso, H. D., Lopez-Jimenez, F., Buring, J. E., & Gaziano, J. M. (2004). Alcohol consumption and cardiovascular disease mortality in hypertensive men. *Archives of Internal Medicine, 164*(6), 623-628.

Mayo Clinic staff. (2011). Nutrition and healthy eating - Alcohol use: If you drink, keep it moderate. Retrieved January 21, 2010, from http://www.mayoclinic.com /health/alcohol/SC00024

Mokdad, A. H., Marks, J. S., Stroup, D. F., & Gerberding, J. L. (2004). Actual causes of death in the United States, 2000. *Journal of the American Medical Association, 291,* 1238-1245.

Mukamal, K. J., Maclure, M., Muller, J. E., Sherwood, J. B., & Mittleman, M. A. (2001). Prior alcohol consumption and mortality following acute myocardial infarction. *Journal of the American Medical Association, 285,* 1965-1970.

Muntwyler, J., Hennekens, C. H., Buring, J. E., & Gaziano, J. M. (1998). Mortality and light to moderate alcohol consumption after myocardial infarction. Lancet, *352,* 1882-1885.

Naimi, T. S., Brewer, R. D., Mokdad, A., Denny, C., & Serdula, M. K. (2003). Binge drinking among U.S. adults. *Journal of the American Medical Association, 289,* 70-75.

National Council on Alcoholism and Drug Dependence. (n.d.). History and mission. Retrieved May 26, 2011, from http:// www.ncadd.org/history/events.html

National Heart, Blood, & Lung Institute. (2010). Heart failure:

What is heart failure? Retrieved April 14, 2011, from http://www.nhlbi.nih.gov/health/dci/Diseases/Hf/HF_WhatIs.html

National Highway Traffic Safety Administration. (2001). *The traffic stop & you: Improving communications between citizens and law enforcement* (Publication No. DOT HS 809 212). Retrieved from http://www.nhtsa.dot.gov/people/injury/enforce /Traffic%20 Stop%20&%20You%20HTML/TrafficStop_index.htm

National Highway Traffic Safety Administration. (2009). *Traffic safety facts - Research note: Fatal crashes involving young drivers* (Publication No. DOT HS 811 218). Retrieved from http://www-nrd.nhtsa.dot.gov/Pubs/811218.PDF

National Highway Traffic Safety Administration. (2012). *Traffic safety fact: A compilation of motor vehicle crash data from the fatality analysis reporting system and the general estimates system* (Publication No. DOT HS 811 659). Retrived from http://www-nrd.nhtsa.dot.gov/Pubs/811659.

National Institute on Alcohol Abuse and Alcoholism. (n.d.). Facts about alcohol poisoning. Retrieved September 10, 2010, from http://www.collegedrinkingprevention.gov / OtherAlcoholInformation/factsAboutAlcoholPoisoning.aspx

National Institute on Alcohol Abuse and Alcoholism. (1993). *Alcohol alert: Alcohol and cancer* (No. 21 PH 345). Rockville, MD: Author.

National Institute on Alcohol Abuse and Alcoholism. (2000) *Alcohol Alert: Fetal alcohol exposure and the brain* (No. 50). Retrieved from http://pubs.niaaa.nih.gov /publications/aa50. htm

National Institute on Alcohol Abuse and Alcoholism. (2004, Winter). NIAAA Council Approves Definition of Binge

Drinking. *NIAA Newsletter.* Retrieved September 12, 2010 from http://www.niaaa.nih.gov

National Institute on Drug Abuse. (n.d.a). Alcohol. Retrieved September 12, 2010, from http://www.nida.nih.gov/DrugPages/ Alcohol.html

National Institute on Drug Abuse. (n.d.b). *Prescription drugs: Abuse and addiction* (Research Report Series). Retrieved from http://www.nida.nih.gov/ResearchReports/Prescription / prescription3.html#CNS

National Institute on Drug Abuse. (2003). *Preventing drug use among children and adolescents: A research-based guide for parents, educators, and community leaders* (2nd ed.). Retrieved from http://www.drugabuse.gov/pdf/prevention/RedBook. pdf

National Institute on Drug Abuse. (2005). *Heroin: Abuse and addiction* (Research Report Series, NIH Publication No. 05-4165). Retrieved from http://www.drugabuse.gov /PDF/ RRHeroin.pdf

National Institute on Drug Abuse. (2008). *Drugs, brains, and behavior - The science of addiction* (NIH Publication No. 07-5605). Bethesda, MD: Author.

National Institute on Drug Abuse. (2009). *NIDA infofacts: Prescription and over-the-counter medications.* Retrieved from http://www.drugabuse.gov/Infofacts/PainMed.html

National Institute on Drug Abuse. (2010a). *Cocaine: Abuse and addiction* (Research Report Series). Retrieved from http://www. drugabuse.gov/ResearchReports/Cocaine /Cocaine.html

National Institute on Drug Abuse. (2010b). *Inhalant Abuse* (Research

Report Series, NIH Publication No. 09-3818). Retrieved from http://www.nida.nih.gov/PDF/RRinhalants.pdf

National Institute on Drug Abuse. (2010c). *NIDA infofacts: Club drugs (GHB, ketamine and Rohypnol)*. Retrieved from http://www.drugabuse.gov/infofacts/clubdrugs.html

National Institute on Drug Abuse. (2011). Marijuana: An update from the National Institute on Drug Abuse. Retrieved from http://www.nida.nih.gov/tib/marijuana.html

New York City Department of Health and Mental Hygiene. (2009). Health department report links heavy drinking to increased risk of HIV and other STDs. Retrieved from http://www.nyc.gov/html/doh/html/pr2009/pr001-09.shtml

Pope, H. G., & Yurgelun-Todd, D. (1996). The residual cognitive effects of heavy marijuana use in college students. *Journal of the American Medical Association, 275*(7), 521-527.

Reinberg, S. (2007, May 2). Drinking Shrinks the Brain. *HealthDay News*. Retrieved from http://www.healthscout.com/template.asp?page=newsdetail&ap=1&id=604213

Sarafian, T. A., Magallanes, J. A., Shau, H., Tashkin, D., & Roth, M. D. (1999). Oxidative stress produced by marijuana smoke: An adverse effect enhanced by cannabinoids. *American Journal of Respiratory Cell and Molecular Biology, 20*(6), 1286-1293.

Scheier, L. M., & Botvin, G. J. (1996). Effects of early adolescent drug use on cognitive efficacy in early-late adolescence: A developmental structural model. *Journal of Substance Abuse, 7*(4), 397-404.

Scott, K. D., Schafer, J., & Greenfield, T. K. (1999). The role of alcohol in physical assault perpetration and victimization. *Journal of Studies on Alcohol, 60*, 528-536.

Solomon, C. G., Frank, B., Hu, F. B, Stampfer, M. J., Colditz, G. A., Speizer, F. E., . . . Manson, J. E. (2000). Moderate alcohol consumption and risk of coronary heart disease among women with type 2 diabetes mellitus. Circulation, *102*, 494-499.

Substance Abuse and Mental Health Services Administration, Office of Applied Studies. (2004). *Results from the 2003 National Survey on Drug Use and Health: National findings* (NSDUH Series H-25, HHS Publication No. SMA 04-3964). Rockville, MD: Author.

Substance Abuse and Mental Health Services Administration, Office of Applied Studies. (2007). *Results from the 2006 National Survey on Drug Use and Health: National findings* (NSDUH Series H-32, HHS Publication No. SMA 07-4293).Retrieved from http://oas.samhsa.gov/nsduh/2k6nsduh/2k6results.cfm

Substance Abuse and Mental Health Services Administration, Office of Applied Studies. (2008). *Results from the 2007 National Survey on Drug Use and Health: National findings* (NSDUH Series H-34, HHS Publication No. SMA 08-4343). Rockville, MD: Author.

Substance Abuse and Mental Health Services Administration, Office of Applied Studies. (2009a). *The NSDUH Report: Marijuana use and perceived risk of use among adolescents: 2002 to 2007.* Retrieved from http://oas.samhsa.gov/2k9/Mjrisks /MJrisks.pdf

Substance Abuse and Mental Health Services Administration, Office of Applied Studies. (2009b). *Results from the 2008 National Survey on Drug Use and Health: National findings* (NSDUH Series H-36, HHS Publication No. SMA 09-4434). Rockville, MD: Author.

Thadhani, R., Camargo, C. A., Jr., Stampfer, M. J., Curhan, G. C.,Willett, W. C., & Rimm, E. B. (2002). Prospective study of moderate alcohol consumption and risk of hypertension in young women. *Archives of Internal Medicine, 162*(5), 569-574.

U.S. Department of Health and Human Services. (2000). *Healthy People 2010* (2nd ed.). Washington, DC: Government Printing Office.

U.S. Department of Health and Human Services. (2007). *The Surgeon General's call to action to prevent and reduce underage drinking: A guide to action for educators.* Retrieved from http://www.surgeongeneral.gov/topics/underagedrinking/educatorguide.pdf

U.S. Department of Health and Human Services & U.S. Department of Agriculture. (2008). Alcoholic Beverages. In *Dietary guidelines for Americans, 2005* (6th ed.). Retrieved March 28, 2010, from http://www.health.gov/DIETARYGUIDELINES/dga2005 /document/html/chapter9.htm

U.S. Department of Justice. (2000). *Promising strategies to reduce substance abuse* (Publication No. NCJ 183152). Retrieved from http://www.ncjrs.gov/pdffiles1/ojp/183152.pdf

Volkow, N. (2005). Letter from the Director. In *Marijuana Abuse* (Research report series, NIH Publication No. 10-3859). Retrieved from http://www.drugabuse.gov/ResearchReports /Marijuana/default.html

Volkow, N. (2011, September 22). Congressional caucus on prescription drug abuse. Testimony to U.S. Congress. Retrieved from http://www.nida.nih.gov/Testimony/9-22-10Testimony.html

World Health Organization. (2007). *Alcohol and injury in emergency departments: Summary of the report from the WHO Collaborative Study on Alcohol and Injuries.* Retrieved from http://www.who.int/substance_abuse/publications /alcohol_injury_summary.pdf

TOBACCO

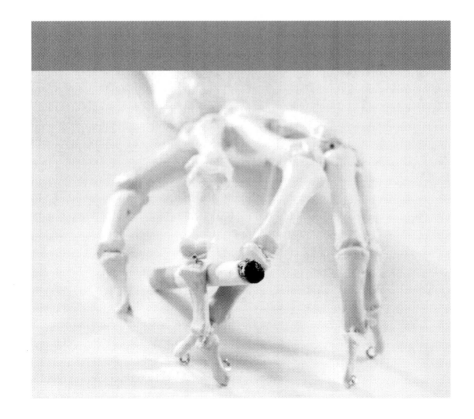

Tobacco use is one of the leading preventable contributors to disease, disability, and death in the United States, and it is the single most preventable cause of death in the world today (World Health Organization [WHO], 2008). Between 1964 and 2004, cigarette smoking caused an estimated 12 million deaths, including 4.1 million deaths from cancer, 5.5 million deaths from cardiovascular diseases, 1.1 million deaths from respiratory diseases, and 94,000 infant deaths related to mothers smoking during pregnancy (U.S. Department of Health and Human Services [HHS], 2004). According to the Centers for Disease Control and Prevention (CDC, 2008a), cigarette smoking results in more than 400,000 premature deaths in the United States each year, or about 1 in every 5 U.S. deaths. Tobacco is the only legal consumer product that can harm everyone who comes into contact with it, and it kills up to half of those who use it as intended. More people die from using tobacco than from alcohol and drug use, fires, motor vehicle accidents, suicides, homicides, and AIDS combined (Patkar, Vergare, Batra, Weinstein, & Leone, 2003).

The past two decades have seen major tobacco-use control efforts and successful campaigns to establish an informed public regarding the dangers of tobacco. Despite these strides, approximately 23.3% of Americans continue to smoke (CDC, 2002). The tobacco industry is a partial contributor to new-smoker initiation with its continued promotions targeting "replacement smokers" to supplant the individuals that have quit smoking or have died (WHO, 2008). Reports from the Institute of Medicine (IOM) warn that, in spite of the downward trend in tobacco use since 1964, current smoking trends indicate the annual smoking cessation rate is still somewhat low. Also, the decline in smoking initiation has slowed down and the overall adult smoking rate appears to be flattening out around 20%. These trends show that a substantial amount of effort will be needed to address this continuing health crisis (IOM, 2007). Reports from the CDC maintain that approximately 80% of adult smokers started smoking before the age of 18 years. Moreover, each day in the United States about 4,000 young people try smoking and 1,140 young people become daily smokers. If the current smoking trends persist, roughly 5 million youth will eventually die prematurely of tobacco-related diseases. In addition, nearly 70% of the 45.3 million Americans who smoke *want* to quit but cannot (CDC, 2008c).

Types of Tobacco Exposure

Nicotine can be introduced into the body by various means. Although cigarettes are the most common, tobacco comes in many forms and all are harmful. The discussion in this section is limited to the more common forms of tobacco exposure other than cigarettes: cigars, pipes, smokeless tobacco, and second-hand smoke.

Cigars

Cigars go through a different manufacturing process than cigarettes, which results in a different kind of tobacco. This does not mean that they are safer. In fact, cigar smoke is as or more toxic and carcinogenic than cigarette smoke. Most types of cancer caused by cigarette smoking are detected at higher rates among regular cigar smokers. Also, those who inhale deeply while smoking a cigar and who smoke several cigars a day experience higher rates of coronary heart disease and chronic obstructive pulmonary disease (Burns, 1998).

Pipes

Pipe smoking was in steady decline from the mid 1960's until recently. The decline was most likely due to such factors as lack of appeal to the younger generations and lack of marketing by tobacco companies. Due to the decline in pipe use, deaths attributable to pipe use have also declined (Nelson, Davis, Chrismon, & Giovino, 1996). However, some recent evidence indicates it may be catching on with the "twenty-something" crowd. Pipe tobacco sales appear to be on the rise, possibly due to a new demographic of young pipe smokers. As cigarettes become more and more expensive, pipe tobacco is being marketed as a cheaper alternative (Pilon, 2009). Another trend with young people is waterpipes, also known by such names as argileh, goza, hookah, shisha, and hubble-bubble. The most common type of tobacco used with this type of pipe is flavored and sweetened (Noonan & Kulbok, 2009). A common misconception is that smoking tobacco from a waterpipe is less harmful. Waterpipe smoke can contain high levels of toxic compounds like carbon monoxide, heavy metals, and cancer-causing chemicals (Sajid, Akhter, & Malik, 1993; Shihadeh & Saleh, 2005).

Smokeless Tobacco

There are two main types of smokeless tobacco in the United States: chew and snuff (Federal Trade Commission, 2009). Smokeless tobacco products are different than other tobacco products in their composition and chemical profile; however, these products still contain the addictive substance nicotine. The amount of nicotine in smokeless tobacco products is manipulated during the manufacturing process, and nicotine levels vary by brand. Smokeless tobacco contains a number of known carcinogens that cause health problems. Multiple studies have found it to cause different types of cancer, such as oral cancer, throat cancer, and pancreatic cancer (International Agency for Research on Cancer [IARC], 2007).

Secondhand Smoke

Research confirms that involuntarily inhaling tobacco smoke results in increased risk of health problems for non-smokers (HHS, 2006). It is estimated that secondhand smoke causes 46,000 premature deaths from heart disease each year (CDC, 2008b). Exposure to secondhand smoke at home or work can increase the risk of developing heart disease by 25%-30% in non-smokers. Secondhand smoke can increase the risk of heart attack because breathing the smoke interferes with the regular functioning of blood and blood vessels. People already suffering from heart problems are at an even greater risk for health issues from secondhand smoke (HHS, 2006). Annually, approximately 3,400 non-smokers die from lung cancer in the United States (CDC, 2008b). Secondhand smokers inhale the same chemicals and poison that smokers inhale. Secondhand smoke contains more than 50 cancer-causing chemicals and even brief exposure can have detrimental effects on cells and put the cancer process in motion. Exposure to it in the womb and in the home has also been shown to contribute to Sudden Infant Death Syndrome (HHS, 2006).

Biology and Physiology

In addition to environmental and behavioral factors, genetic and physiological components influence smoking habits. The study of genetic influence on smoking behavior is still in its infancy, but it is showing promise in identifying the particular genes that contribute to smoking initiation, addiction, and cessation. Some studies have demonstrated that smoking is as heritable as alcoholism and some mental disorders, such as schizophrenia (Carmelli, Swan, Robinette, & Fabsitz, 1992; Edwards, Austin, and Jarvik, 1995; Heath et al., 1993; Kendler et al., 1999; Schnoll, Johnson, & Lerman, 2007; True et al., 1997).

Many physiological reactions occur when nicotine is introduced into one's body. When smoke is inhaled from a cigarette, the nicotine is taken from the tobacco, carried to the lungs in the smoke, absorbed rapidly into the bloodstream, and then moved quickly to the brain. Many harm-causing toxic chemicals are in cigarettes, but nicotine is the component that causes the actual physical addiction to smoking (Benowitz, 2008a, 2008b). The nicotine is what hooks an individual and creates dependence. Nicotine facilitates the release of chemicals, such as dopamine, that make one feel good and produces the feeling of pleasure. After repeated exposure to nicotine, the brain becomes accustomed to the nicotine and builds up a tolerance to the many effects of the chemical. Then, when someone tries to quit, they experience withdrawal. Withdrawal is characterized by irritability, anxiety, increased eating, depression, and other unpleasant symptoms. Smoking is also reinforced by other stimuli, such as the smell of a cigarette or other associations with smoking that the smoker may have, like having a cocktail or being in social situations with other smokers (Benowitz, 2008a, 2008b). Around 80% of smokers would like to quit, but only about 5% have been successful quitting on their own. This is mostly due to the extremely addictive nature of nicotine (Baille, Mattick, & Hall, 1995).

Sociocultural Influences

The initiation of using tobacco has many antecedents. Multiple factors contribute to one's choice of vices. Becoming addicted to nicotine products usually involves a process. Typically, the first time an individual tries a cigarette it is experimental and out of curiosity. Peer pressure is also a very influential factor that impacts young individuals and their choice to begin smoking. For example, about 38% of middle school students and 25% of high school students believe that smokers have more friends (Eaton et al., 2006). Statistics indicate that 54% of high school students have at least tried smoking and that 16% of high school students have smoked a whole cigarette by the age of 13 years old (Lantz et al., 2000). The median age for trying cigarettes is 15 years old (CDC, 2001). Adolescence is a prime time to become addicted to nicotine because those who try smoking during this important developmental stage are at a greater risk of becoming daily smokers by the age of 18 years old (Breslau & Peterson, 1996; Elders, Perry, Eriksen, & Giovino, 1994; Escobedo, Marcus, Holtzman, & Giovino, 1993), and they are less likely to eventually stop smoking (Cleary, Hitchcock, Semmer, Flinchbaugh, & Pinney, 1988; Daniel, Johnston, & Levy, 1981).

The tobacco industry deliberately targets young adults aged 18-24 years. Young adults in particular are believed to be influenced by media and marketing in addition to being old enough to buy tobacco products (*Conjoint Simulation Model*, 1993; Ling & Glantz, 2002; Mowery, Brick, Farrelly, 2000). Tobacco companies use detailed studies of young adult behavior and pertinent environmental influences to guide their marketing and advertising strategies (Potter, Pederson, Chan, Aubut, & Koval, 2004). In addition to the machinations of the tobacco industry, individuals are also susceptible to aspects of social pressure, such as body image. Maintaining a socially acceptable body shape is one of the many influential determinants of smoking behavior (Steptoe & Wardle, 2004). Young women are often vulnerable to this brand of societal pressure and tend to be more likely than men to use smoking for weight control and weight loss (Boles & Johnson, 2001; Stice & Shaw, 2003) because they are more likely than male smokers to *believe* smoking is a way to control weight (Rossow & Rise, 1994). Young women also possess a greater likelihood for smoking more regularly than young men and finding it more difficult to quit smoking (Ellickson, Tucker, & Klein, 2001; Lowry, Guluska, & Fulton, 2002).

Other environmental and social factors contribute to an individual's proclivity to initiate tobacco use. Growing up with parents who are smokers potentially predisposes children toward becoming daily smokers when they grow older (Rossow & Rise, 1994). This predisposition is thought to be caused by at least three things: (1) biological vulnerability to tobacco, such as genetic factors and exposure to nicotine in utero and during childhood; (2) modeling of parental behavior; and (3) tolerant attitudes toward smoking in the individual's family (Kestilä et al., 2006). Education level of parents can also help determine whether someone starts using tobacco. The less education parents have, the more likely they are to smoke and then influence their children to smoke. However, this can be mediated by one's own education: As an individual becomes more educated, they are less likely to smoke (2006).

Smoking rates and incidence rates of smoking-related lung cancer reflect racial and ethnic disparities in the United States. Studies comparing Whites, Blacks, Native Hawaiians/other Polynesians,

Japanese Americans, and Latinos have demonstrated that the incidence of lung cancer is much higher among Blacks and Native Hawaiians/other Polynesians than among Whites. However, lung cancer rates were lower among Japanese Americans and Latinos than the other groups (HHS, 1998). Smoking behavior also varies among these highlighted ethnic and racial groups. For example, 30.1% of Black adults smoke cigarettes compared to 27.3 % of White adults. Interestingly, only 8% of Black smokers reported being heavy smokers (smoking at least 25 cigarettes per day) as compared to 28.3% of White smokers. Although Black smokers tend to smoke fewer cigarettes, they take in 30% more nicotine than Whites (Perez-Stable, Herrera, Jacob, & Benowitz, 1998). Native Hawaiians have higher rates of lung cancer than Whites and Asians, even though the smoking habits of these groups are alike (Kolonel, 1979; Menck & Henderson, 1982). Menthol cigarettes are also a factor that contributes to racial and ethnic differences in smoking behavior. Research indicates that menthol cigarettes are more harmful and create more difficulty when trying to quit. The most frequent users of menthol cigarettes are African Americans. Seventy-five percent of African American smokers choose to smoke menthol cigarettes as opposed to 20%-30% of White Americans (Pletcher et al., 2006).

Not all tobacco users struggle with nicotine addiction. Some individuals enjoy a cigarette on occasion or smoke lightly (less than 5 cigarettes a day) but do not fit the criteria for nicotine dependence (APA, 2000). Some individuals will smoke cigarettes under particular situations, such as after a meal, while drinking alcohol, or with particular friends. Although these smokers may not experience the nicotine withdrawal that daily smokers endure, it is a type of dependence and could have possible negative effects (Coggins, Murrelle, Carchman, & Heidbreder, 2009).

Treatment

Currently, the most common methods to aid smokers in quitting the habit are nicotine- replacement products and pharmaceutical agents, such as bupropion (market name Zyban) and varenicline (market name Chantix). Nicotine-replacement products include the transdermal patch, gum, intranasal spray, vapor inhaler, lozenge, and sublingual tablet (Shiffman, Mason, & Henningfield, 1998). For smokers, nicotine addiction is created and sustained by the spike in nicotine levels in the bloodstream generated by inhaling cigarette smoke. Unfortunately, nicotine-replacement therapies do not provide the same kind of nicotine spike as actually smoking a cigarette. However, they do provide a therapeutic level of nicotine that has been shown to be effective for some people (Vaszar, Sarinas, & Lillington, 2002).

Varenicline and bupropion are on the list of recommended first-line smoking cessation medications in the U.S. Public Health Service's clinical practice guidelines (National Cancer Institute, 2009). Bupropion, or Zyban, is an atypical anti-depressant and is the only non-nicotine product approved as a first line of therapy for quitting smoking. It is not completely clear why bupropion works for smoking cessation, but it may be related to the properties of the drug that influence mood and nicotine absorption (Siu & Tyndale, 2007). Varenicline, or Chantix, is the first of a new class of pharmacological methods intended for smoking cessation. The drug was designed to address both the positive reinforcing effects of nicotine and its withdrawal symptoms. Basically, it helps people stop smoking by acting the same way nicotine acts in the brain (Hays, Ebbert, & Sood, 2009).

In response to the reported adverse effects of varenicline and buproprion, the U.S. Food and Drug Administration (FDA) now requires "black box" warning labels on the packaging for the two drugs. The warnings caution users of the drugs about their risks, such as neurological problems, hostility, agitation, depression, suicidal thoughts, suicidal behavior, and suicide attempts. The FDA review noted that these symptoms have occurred in individuals with no history of such issues. The review also documented that some symptoms experienced by users may be confused with the typical symptoms of nicotine withdrawal (National Cancer Institute, 2009).

Therapeutic behavioral treatments have also been found to be effective for smoking cessation and can be administered in various forms. There are four main types of behavioral treatments: (1) minimal advice from a healthcare worker, (2) individual counseling, (3) group counseling, and (4) telephone counseling (Mottillo et al., 2009). These treatments are based on conditioning and the belief that smoking is a learned behavior. Here, methods are employed to unlearn the smoking habit and take away the stimuli or replace it with other things that will help keep a smoker away from the nicotine source (Haustein & Groneberg, 2009). Studies have demonstrated that the more intensive treatments—individual, group, and telephone counseling— contributed to higher rates of cessation when compared to no treatment at all (Lemmens, Oenema, Knut, & Brug, 2008; Mottillo et al., 2009). Current guidelines for smoking cessation include the recommendation to use pharmacological interventions in conjunction with behavioral therapies because this method has been shown to be more effective (Fiore et al., 2008; Lancaster, Stead, Silagy, & Sowden, 2000; Tobacco Use and Dependence Clinical Practice Guideline Panel, Staff, and Consortium Representatives, 2000).

Self-Help for Tobacco Cessation
Most smokers try to quit on their own and prefer using the self-help approach without any formal aid or treatment (Fiore et al., 1990; Glynn, Boyd, & Gruman, 1990). Self-help approaches to quitting smoking can take several forms, ranging from completely unaided attempts to more elaborate but still self-administered programs (Lichtenstein & Cohen, 1990). The various interventions can include pamphlets, manuals, videos, DVDs, internet resources, chat rooms, support groups, books, and, of course, "cold turkey." The many different resources can make being a consumer of tobacco-cessation products complicated. Individuals need to take into consideration

several factors if they decide to quit on their own. Unfortunately, no comprehensive evaluation of all the different self-help methods exists (Curry, 1993; Glynn et al., 1990), making it difficult for consumers to know what will work for them and what will not.

For some, making the decision to quit smoking is very daunting and anxiety provoking, and following through can be an intense struggle. Therefore, choosing the method to quit that best fits with one's specific needs is imperative for success. Some current research asserts that successful cessation interventions must incorporate individual factors like demographics, behavioral characteristics, and living and work environments (Lee & Kahende, 2007). For example, if individuals are trying to quit and they are surrounded by smokers in the home or work place, quitting may be more difficult. Having others' support in different environments can be very helpful toward a successful cessation. Other factors influencing successful cessation include being aged 35 years or older, having a college education, being married or living with a partner, and not switching to low-tar or low-nicotine cigarettes when attempting to quit (2007).

One study examining the use of self-help materials versus the use of no intervention concluded that people using self-help materials do have a better chance of quitting than if they use nothing at all. Also, the study found that using personalized self-help materials was much more helpful and resulted in higher quit rates than using non-personalized materials (Lancaster & Stead, 2005). There is a movement in self-help research toward promoting more tailored and personalized materials (Curry, 1993; Haustein & Groneberg, 2009). Given all the factors that go into determining which self-help method to choose when contemplating quitting tobacco, it is important for people who choose this method to do some research and find the materials that will fit with their lifestyles. If possible, they should discover methods that can be tailored to their specific needs and make sure that they have adequate environmental and social support.

Determining the actual effectiveness of self-help methods can be difficult. Not all methods have been evaluated for efficacy, but, again, it is important to find a method that suits personal needs. For many, self-help materials are the most cost-effective method for quitting the use of tobacco products. Currently, only about one third of insurance companies will cover the cost of smoking-cessation methods (Fuhrmans, 2005). Medications and nicotine-replacement therapies can be expensive and many are unable to pay for these methods on their own. It is important to keep in mind that the one-time purchase of tobacco products is going to be much less than a doctor's visit or medication (Shiffman et al., 1998). Unfortunately, tobacco products are much more accessible than methods for quitting. One study observed a group of people who had insurance that covered tobacco-cessation treatments to see if the quit rates of those covered by insurance exceeded those without insurance coverage. The study found that full coverage of treatment showed to be an effective and relatively low-cost strategy for significantly increasing quit rates, quit attempts, and the use of nicotine gum and the nicotine patch (Schauffler et al., 2001). Unfortunately, many individuals do not have the luxury of full coverage for treatment from their insurance companies. Therefore, self-help materials may be the only viable choice for them.

Complementary and Alternative Medicine (CAM) for Tobacco Cessation

The use of alternative and complementary treatments may be an option to aid tobacco cessation. In a survey conducted in the United States with 31,000 patients, 74.6% of the adults reported using some form of complementary and alternative medicine (Barnes, Powell-Griner, McFann, & Nahin, 2004). Complementary and alternative medicine (CAM) is classified into five groups: (1) alternative medical systems, (2) mind-body interventions, (3) biologically based therapies, (4) manipulative and body-based methods, and (5) energy therapies. These categories include practices such as acupuncture, meditation, hypnosis, massage, relaxation, and herbal products. These methods and products can be used in conjunction with clinical and self-help methods or on their own. Studies have been done on the efficacy of different types of CAM treatments, such as hypnosis, the herbal products Avena sativa and lobeline, mint snuff, black pepper extract, herbal tea preparation, self-massage, transcranial magnetic stimulation, relaxation imagery, urinary alkalization, and tape suggestion under anesthesia. Available evidence does not support the use of any of these interventions for successful tobacco cessation (Sood, Ebbert, Sood, & Stevens, 2006). However, CAM methods may be beneficial by aiding the process in other ways.

CAM methods can help relieve some withdrawal symptoms and provide individuals with skills to aid their cessation (Van Haselen & Friedrich, 2003). For example, one study found that self-massage in conjunction with other cessation methods helped to alleviate smoking-related anxiety, reduced cravings and withdrawal symptoms, improved mood, and, for some, reduced the number of cigarettes they smoked (Hernandez-Reif, Field, & Hart, 1999). Given the complex nature of smoking cessation, the best practice may be to tackle the problem from multiple angles. Although little research shows that CAM methods help people quit tobacco, some evidence indicates that these methods in conjunction with others can be helpful in alleviating a number of the symptoms that accompany quitting (Van Haselen & Friedrich, 2003).

Prevention

Because the majority of smokers start smoking before the age of 18 years, current preventative practices are mostly aimed at young people (Institute of Medicine, 2007). Tobacco- industry campaigns target youth with the intention of hooking them on tobacco products for life (Ling & Glantz, 2002). In response, prevention efforts include media campaigns to counteract the tobacco-industry efforts, school tobacco-prevention programs, and other efforts such as raising the prices of tobacco products and placing them in less accessible areas (Task Force on Community Preventive Services, 2005). Also, smoking bans in the workplace and in public places have been shown to be an effective tool for prevention, and they limit exposure to environmental tobacco smoke for many citizens (Lee & Kahende, 2007).

Conclusion

There are many reasons individuals pick up the habit in spite of the known risks and consequences. Age, gender, genetics, family, environment, and a myriad of other factors influence the decision to use tobacco. Health professionals, researchers, worldwide organizations, and policymakers make continued attempts to prevent new tobacco users and encourage current tobacco users to quit. The preventable nature of tobacco-related illnesses is one of the more perplexing issues in terms of creating and implementing effective interventions. Modern medical advances have reduced or eradicated the majority of communicable diseases responsible for death throughout much of history. However, chronic diseases caused by lifestyle-related behaviors, such as the use of tobacco, are different in nature and modern medicine has not found effective interventions to stave off the consequences of these types of behaviors.

Recommendations

The U.S. Department of Health and Human Services (Fiore et al., 2008) provides the following reasons and impetus for quitting tobacco and makes these recommendations to individuals who are attempting cessation:

Good Reasons for Quitting
You will feel better.
- You will have more energy and breathe easier.
- Your chances of getting sick will go down.

Smoking is dangerous.
- More than 435,000 Americans die each year from smoking.

- Smoking causes illnesses such as cancer, heart disease, stroke, problems with pregnancy, and lung disease.

More Good Reasons for Quitting
If you are pregnant, your baby will be healthier.
- Your baby will get more oxygen.

The people around you, especially children, will be healthier.
- Breathing in other people's smoke can cause asthma and other health problems.

You will have more money. If you smoke one pack per day, quitting smoking could save you up to $150 a month.

Savings Per Month

If you smoke (packs per day)	You pay (per day)	Quitting saves (per month)
1	$5.00	$150
2	$10.00	$300
3	$15.00	$450

There Has Never Been a Better Time to Quit
A combination works best.
- Set a quit date.
- Get support.
- Take medicine.

Get Ready
Get Help
Get Medicine
Stay Quit!

Get Ready
Set a quit date.

No smoking after: _____

Change the things around you.
- Get rid of all cigarettes and ashtrays in your home, car, and place of work.
- Do not let people smoke in your home.

After you quit, don't smoke—not even a puff! Don't use any tobacco!

Get Medicine
You can buy nicotine gum, the nicotine patch, or the nicotine lozenge at a drug store.

You can ask your pharmacist for more information.

Ask your doctor about other medicines that can help you.
- Nicotine nasal spray
- Nicotine inhaler
- Bupropion SR (pill)
- Varenicline (pill)

Most health insurance will pay for these medicines.

Get Help
Tell your family, friends, and people you work with that you are going to quit. Ask for their support.

Talk to your doctor, nurse, or other health care worker. They can help you quit.

Call 1-800-QUIT NOW (784-8669) to be connected to the quitline in your state.

It's free. They will set up a quit plan with you.

Stay Quit
If you "slip" and smoke or chew tobacco, don't give up. Try again soon. Set a new quit date to get back on track.

Avoid alcohol.

Avoid being around smoking.

Eat healthy food and get exercise.

Keep a positive attitude. You **can** do it!

You Can Quit
Most people try several times before they quit for good. Quitting is hard, but—**You Can Quit.**

Selected Resources

American College Health Association
891 Elkridge Landing Road, Suite 100
Linthicum, MD 21090
410-859-1500; Fax: 410-859-1510
www.acha.org/info_resources/ATOD_resources.cfm

Centers for Disease Control and Prevention (CDC)
1600 Clifton Rd.
Atlanta, GA 30333
800-CDC-INFO (800-232-4636); TTY: 888-232-6348
www.cdc.gov/tobacco/
www.cdc.gov/tobacco/quit_smoking/how_to_quit/index.htm

Tobacco.org
P.O. Box 359, Village Station
New York, NY 10014-0359
212-982-4645
www.tobacco.org/resources/general/tobsites.html

TTB.gov
Alcohol and Tobacco Trade Bureau
U.S. Department of the Treasury
www.ttb.gov/consumer/index.shtml

World Health Organization (WHO) Tobacco Free Initiative
Noncommunicable Diseases and Mental Health
Avenue Appia 20
1211 Geneva 27
Switzerland
Fax: + 41 22 791 4832
tfi@who.int
www.who.int/tobacco/en/

References

American Psychiatric Association. (2000). *Diagnostic and statistical manual of mental disorders* (Rev. 4th ed.). Washington, DC: Author.

Baille, A. J., Mattick, R. P., & Hall, W. (1995). Quitting smoking: Estimation by meta-analysis of the rate of unaided smoking cessation. *Australian Journal of Public Health, 19*, 129-131.

Barnes, P. M., Powell-Griner, E., McFann, K., & Nahin, R. L. (2004). Complementary and alternative medicine use among adults: United States, 2002. *Advance Data, 343*, 1-19.

Benowitz, N. L. (2008a). Clinical pharmacology of nicotine: Implications for understanding, preventing, and treating tobacco addiction. *Clinical Pharmacology & Therapeutics, 83*(4), 531-541.

Benowitz, N. L. (2008b). Neurobiology of nicotine addiction: Implications for smoking cessation treatment. *The American Journal of Medicine, 121*(4A), S3-S10.

Boles, S. M., & Johnson, P. B. (2001). Gender, weight concerns, and adolescent smoking. *Journal of Addictive Diseases, 20*(2), 5-14.

Breslau, N., & Peterson, E. L. (1996). Smoking cessation in young adults: Age at initiation of cigarette smoking and other suspected influences. *American Journal of Public Health, 86*(2), 214-220.

Burns, D. (1998). Cigar smoking: Overview and current state of the science. In *Cigars: Health effects and trends. NCI tobacco control monograph 9* (NIH Publication No. 98-4302). Bethesda,

MD: U.S. Department of Health and Human Services, National Institutes of Health, National Cancer Institute.

Carmelli, D., Swan, G. E., Robinette, D., & Fabsitz, R. (1992). Genetic influence on smoking: A study of male twins. *New England Journal of Medicine, 327*(12), 829-833.

Centers for Disease Control and Prevention. (2001). Youth tobacco surveillance: United States, 2000. *Morbidity and Mortality Weekly Report, 50*, SS-04-09.

Centers for Disease Control and Prevention (2002). Cigarette smoking among adults: United States, 2000. *Morbidity and Mortality Weekly Report, 51*, 642-645.

Centers for Disease Control and Prevention. (2008a). *Smoking & tobacco use: Health effects of cigarette smoking.* Retrieved February 22, 2010, from http://www.cdc.gov/tobacco /data_ statistics /fact_sheets/health_effects/effects_cig_smoking/

Centers for Disease Control and Prevention (2008b). Smoking-attributable mortality, years of potential life lost, and productivity losses: United States, 2000-2004. *Morbidity and Mortality Weekly Report, 57*(45), 1226-1228.

Centers for Disease Control and Prevention. (2008c). *Preventing chronic diseases: Investing wisely in health. Preventing tobacco use.* Retrieved from http://www.cdc.gov/nccdphp/publications/ factsheets/Prevention/pdf/tobacco.pdf

Cleary, P. D., Hitchcock, J. L., Semmer, N., Flinchbaugh, L. J., & Pinney, J. M. (1988). Adolescent smoking: Research and health policy. *Milbank Quarterly, 66*(1), 137-171.

Coggins, C. R. E., Murrelle, E. L., Carchman, R. A., & Heidbreder, C. (2009). Light and intermittent cigarette smokers: A review (1989-2009). *Psychopharmacology, 207*, 343-363.

Conjoint simulation model (Bates No. 2045199142/9311). [ca. 1993, February 23]. Retrieved from Philip Morris USA Public Document Site: http://www.pmdocs.com/pdf/2045199142_931 1_55iosqbm5obn0afjajim10bv.pdf

Curry, S. J. (1993). Self-help interventions for smoking cessation. *Journal of Consulting and Clinical Psychology, 61,* 790-803.

Daniel, H. Johnston, M. E., & Levy, C. J. (1981). *8102 Young smokers prevalence, trends, implications, and related demographic trends* (Bates No. 2062811910/2062811958). Retrieved from Philip Morris USA Public Document Site: http://www.pmdocs.com/ pdf /2062811910_2062811958_55iosqbm5obn0afjajim10bv.pdf

Eaton, D. K., Kann, L., Kinchen, S., Ross, J., Hawkins, J., Harris, W. A., . . . Wechsler, H. (2006). Youth risk behavior surveillance: United States, 2005. *Morbidity and Mortality Weekly Report Surveillance Summary, 55*(5), 1-108.

Edwards, K. L., Austin, M. A., & Jarvik, G. P. (1995). Evidence for genetic influences on smoking in adult women twins. *Clinical Genetics, 47*(5), 236-244.

Elders, M. J., Perry, C. L., Eriksen, M. P., & Giovino, G. A. (1994). The report of the Surgeon General: Preventing tobacco use among young people. *American Journal of Public Health, 84*(4), 543-547.

Ellickson, P. L., Tucker, J. S., & Klein, D. J. (2001). Sex differences in predictors of adolescent smoking cessation. *Health Psychology, 20*(3), 186-195.

Escobedo, L. G., Marcus, S. E., Holtzman, D., & Giovino, G. A. (1993). Sports participation, age at smoking initiation, and the risk of smoking among US high school students. *Journal of the American Medical Association, 269*(11), 1391-1395.

Federal Trade Commission. (2009). *Federal Trade Commission smokeless tobacco report for the year 2006*. Retrieved from http://www.ftc.gov/os/2009/08 /090812smokelesstobaccoreport.pdf

Fiore, M. C., Jaén, C. R., Baker, T. B., Bailey, W. C., Benowitz, N. L., Curry, S. J., . . . Wewers, M. E. (2008). *Treating tobacco use and dependence: 2008 update. Clinical Practice Guideline*. Rockville, MD: U.S. Department of Health and Human Services, Public Health Service.

Fiore, M. C., Novotny, T. E., Pierce, J. P., Giovino, G. A., Hatziandreu, E. J., Newcomb, P. A., . . . Davis, R. M. (1990). Methods used to quit smoking in the United States: Do cessation programs help? *Journal of the American Medical Association, 263*(20), 2760-2765.

Fuhrmans, V. (2005, April 26). Case grows to cover quitting. *The Wall Street Journal*, p. D1.

Glynn, J., Boyd, G. M., & Gruman, J. C. (1990). Essential elements of self-help/minimal intervention strategies for smoking cessation. *Health Education Quarterly, 17*(3), 329-345.

Haustein, K. O., & Groneberg, D. (2009). *Tobacco or health? Physiological and social damages caused by tobacco smoking* (2nd ed.). New York, NY: Springer.

Hays, J. T., Ebbert, J. O., & Sood, A. (2009). Treating tobacco dependence in light of the 2008 US Department of Health and Human Services clinical practice guideline. *Mayo Clinic Proceedings, 84*(8), 730-735.

Heath, A. C., Cates, R., Martin, N. G., Mayer, J., Hewitt, J. K., Neale, M. C., & Eaves, L. J. (1993). Genetic contribution to risk of smoking initiation: Comparisons across birth cohorts and across cultures. *Journal of Substance Abuse, 5*(3), 221-246.

Hernandez-Reif, M., Field, T., & Hart, S. (1999). Smoking cravings are reduced by self-massage. *Preventive Medicine, 28*, 28-32.

Institute of Medicine. (2007, May). *Ending the tobacco problem: A blueprint for the nation* (Report brief). Retrieved from www. iom.edu/Reports/2007/Ending-the-Tobacco-Problem-A-Blueprint-for-the-Nation.aspx

International Agency for Research on Cancer. (2007). *Smokeless tobacco and some tobacco-specific N-Nitrosamines (IARC monographs on the evaluation of carcinogenic risks to humans: Vol. 89)*. Retrieved from http://monographs.iarc.fr/ENG/ Monographs /vol89/mono89.pdf

Kendler, K. S., Neale, M. C., Sullivan, P., Corey, L. A., Gardner, C. O., & Prescott, C. A. (1999). A population based twin study in women of smoking initiation and dependence. *Psychological Medicine, 29*, 299-308.

Kestilä, L., Koskinen, S., Martelin, T., Rahkonen, O., Pensola, T., Pirkola, S, . . . Aromaa, A. (2006). Influence of parental education, childhood adversities, and current living conditions on daily smoking in early adulthood. *European Journal of Public Health, 16*(6), 617-626.

Kolonel, L. (1979). Smoking and drinking patterns among different ethnic groups in Hawaii. *National Cancer Institute Monographs, 53*, 81-87.

Lancaster, T., & Stead, L. F. (2005). Self-help interventions for smoking cessation. *Cochrane Database of Systematic Reviews, 3*.

Lancaster, T., Stead, L., Silagy, C., & Sowden, A. (2000). Effectiveness of interventions to help people stop smoking: Findings from the Cochrane Library. *British Medical Journal, 321*, 355-358.

Lantz, P. M., Jacobson, P. D., Warner, K. E., Wasserman, J., Pollack, H. A., Berson, J., & Ahlstrom, A. (2000). Investing in youth tobacco control: A review of smoking prevention and control strategies. *Tobacco Control, 9*(1), 47-63.

Lee, C., & Kahende, J. (2007). Factors associated with successful smoking cessation in the United States, 2000. *American Journal of Public Health, 97*, 1503-1509.

Lemmens, V., Oenema, A., Knut, I. K., & Brug, J. (2008). Effectiveness of smoking cessation interventions among adults: A systematic review of reviews. *European Journal of Cancer Prevention, 17*(6), 535-544.

Lichtenstein, E., & Cohen, S. (1990). Prospective analysis of two modes of unaided smoking cessation. *Health Education Research, 5*, 63-72.

Ling, P., & Glantz, S. (2002). Why and how the tobacco industry sells cigarettes to young adults: Evidence from industry documents. *American Journal of Public Health, 92*, 908-916.

Lowry, R., Guluska, D. A., & Fulton, J. E. (2002). Weight management goals and practices among US high school students: Associations with physical activity, diet and smoking. *Journal of Adolescent Health, 31*, 133-144.

Menck, H. R., & Henderson, B. E. (1982). Cancer incidence patterns in the Pacific Basin. *National Cancer Institute Monographs, 62*, 101-109.

Mottillo, S., Filion, K. B., Bélisle, P., Joseph, L., Gervais, A., O'Loughlin, J., . . . Eisenberg, M. J. (2009). Behavioural interventions for smoking cessation: A meta-analysis of randomized controlled trials. *European Heart Journal, 30*(6), 718-730.

Mowery, P., Brick, P., & Farrelly, M. (2000). *First look report 3: Pathways to established Smoking - Results from the 1999 National Youth Tobacco Survey.* Washington, DC: American Legacy Foundation.

National Cancer Institute. (2009, July). Black box warnings added to two smoking cessation drugs. *National Cancer Institute Bulletin, 6*(14), 8. Retrieved from http://www.cancer.gov/aboutnci/ncicancerbulletin/archive/2009/071409/page8.

Nelson, D. E., Davis, R. M., Chrismon, J. H., & Giovino, J. A. (1996). Pipe smoking in the United States, 1965-1991: Prevalence and attributable mortality. *Preventive medicine, 25,* 91-99.

Noonan, D., & Kulbok, P. A. (2009). New tobacco trends: Waterpipe (hookah) smoking and implications for healthcare providers. *Journal of the American Academy of Nurse Practitioners, 21,* 258-260.

Patkar, A. A., Vergare, M. J., Batra, V., Weinstein, S. P., & Leone, F. T. (2003, Fall). Tobacco smoking: Current concepts in etiology and treatment. *Psychiatry, 66*(3), 183-199.

Perez-Stable, E. J., Herrera, B., Jacob, P., III, & Benowitz, N. L. (1998). Nicotine metabolism and intake in Black and White smokers. *Journal of the American Medical Association 280,* 152-156.

Pilon, M. (2009, February 20). The latest thing they're smoking in pipes on college campuses: Tobacco - Despite risks, more young people light up; 'It looked like the coolest thing ever.' *The Wall Street Journal,* p. A1.

Pletcher, M. J., Hulley, B. J., Houston, T., Kiefe, C. I., Benowitz, N., & Sidney, S. (2006). Menthol cigarettes, smoking cessation, atherosclerosis, and pulmonary function. *Archive of Internal Medicine, 166,* 1915-1922.

Potter, B. K., Pederson, L. L., Chan, S. S. H., Aubut, J. A. L., & Koval, J. J. (2004). Does a relationship exist between body weight, concerns about weight, and smoking among adolescents? An integration of the literature with an emphasis on gender. *Nicotine and Tobacco Research, 6*, 397-425.

Rossow, I., & Rise, J. (1994). Concordance of parental and adolescent health behaviors. *Social Science and Medicine, 38*, 1299-1305.

Sajid, K. M., Akhter, M., & Malik, G. Q. (1993). Carbon monoxide fractions in cigarette and hookah (hubble bubble) smoke. *Journal of the Pakistan Medical Association, 43*(9), 179-182.

Schauffler, H. H., McMenamin, S., Olson, K., Boyce-Smith, G., Rideout, J. A., & Kamil, J. (2001). Variations in treatment benefits influence smoking cessation: Results of a randomized control trial. *Tobacco Control, 10*, 175-180.

Schnoll, R. A., Johnson, T. A., & Lerman, C. (2007). Genetics and smoking behavior. *Current Psychiatry Reports, 9*, 349-357.

Shiffman, S., Mason, K. M., Henningfield, J. E. (1998). Tobacco dependence treatments: Review and prospectus. *Annual Review of Public Health, 19*, 335-358.

Shihadeh, A., & Saleh, R. (2005). Polycyclic aromatic hydrocarbons, carbon monoxide, "tar," and nicotine in the mainstream smoke aerosol of narghile waterpipe. *Food and Chemical Toxicology, 43*, 655-666.

Siu, E. C. K., & Tyndale, R. (2007). Non-nicotinic therapies for smoking cessation. *Annual Review of Pharmacology and Toxicology, 47*, 541-564.

Sood, A., Ebbert, J. O., Sood, R., & Stevens, S. R. (2006). Complementary treatments for tobacco cessation: A survey. *Nicotine and Tobacco Research, 8*(6), 767-771.

Steptoe, A., & Wardle, J. (2004). Health related behaviour: Prevalence and links with disease. In A. Kaptein & J. Weinman (Eds.), *Health psychology* (pp. 21-51). Buckingham, England: Open University Press.

Stice, E., & Shaw, H. (2003). Prospective relations of body image, eating, and affective disturbances to smoking onset in adolescent girls: How Virginia slims. *Journal of Consulting and Clinical Psychology, 71*, 129-135.

Task Force on Community Preventive Services. (2005). Tobacco. In S. Zaza, P. A. Briss, & K. W. Harris (Eds.), *The guide to Community Preventive Services: What works to promote health?* (pp. 3-79). Atlanta, GA: Oxford University Press.

Tobacco Use and Dependence Clinical Practice Guideline Panel, Staff, and Consortium Representatives. (2000). A clinical practice guideline for treating tobacco use and dependence: A U.S. Public Health Service report. *Journal of the American Medical Association, 283*, 3244-3254.

True, W. R., Heath, A. C., Scherrer, J. F., Waterman, B., Goldberg, J., Lin, N., ... Tsuang, M. T. (1997). Genetic and environmental contributions to smoking. *Addiction, 92*(10), 1277-1287.

U.S. Department of Health and Human Services. (1998). *Tobacco use among U.S. racial/ethnic minority groups — African-Americans, American-Indians and Alaska Natives, Asian-Americans and Pacific Islanders, and Hispanics: A report of the Surgeon General.* Atlanta, GA: Centers for Disease Control and Prevention.

U.S. Department of Health and Human Services. (2004). *The health consequences of smoking: what it means to you. The 2004 Surgeon General's report.* Retrieved from http://www.cdc.gov/tobacco/data_statistics/sgr/2004/pdfs/whatitmeanstoyou.pdf

U.S. Department of Health and Human Services. (2006). *The health consequences of involuntary exposure to tobacco smoke: A report of the Surgeon General.* Atlanta, GA: Author.

Van Haselen, R. A., & Friedrich, M. E. (2003). A comprehensive assessment of the role of complementary and alternative medicine in smoking cessation. *Perfusion, 16*(10), 364-369.

Vaszar, L. T., Sarinas, P. S. A., & Lillington, G. A. (2002). Achieving tobacco cessation: Current status, current problems, future possibilities. *Respiration, 69*, 381-384.

World Health Organization. (2008). *WHO report on the global tobacco epidemic, 2008.* Retrieved from http://www.who.int/tobacco/mpower/en/

AGING, DEATH, AND DYING

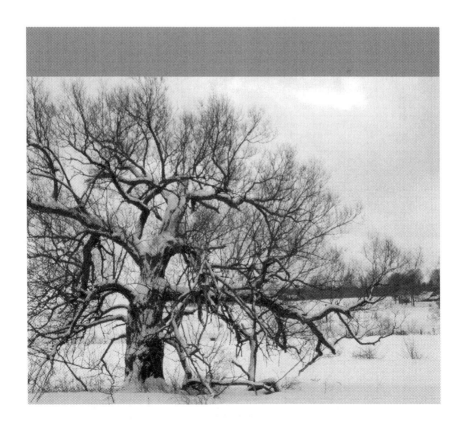

D ue to the Baby Boomer generation entering retirement age and the increase in life expectancy, aging has arrived at the forefront of policy and the concern of U.S. health officials. The nation is entering a period in which the number of older adults has exceeded any known figures throughout history. The current mandate to adequately meet the needs of this population is a challenging one and will have to address issues related to spending and health-care provisions. The face of death is also evolving due to the large aging population, and there has been a demand to return to the practices of past generations. Resources are also becoming increasingly more available to aid families in creating a peaceful and personal environment for themselves and their dying loved ones.

Sociocultural Influences

Modern developments have contributed to a considerable increase in lifespan over recent centuries. At the beginning of the 19th century, life expectancy hovered between 25 and 40 years (Maddison, 2001). From 1900 to 2006, life expectancy at birth increased from 46 to 75 years of age for men, and for women there was an increase from 48 to 80 years old (Fried, 2000). From 1950 through 2006, life expectancy at age 65 for men rose from 13 years to 17 years, and among women it rose from 15 years to 20 years (National Center for Health Statistics, 2009). As industrialization and increased population growth coincided with economic prosperity, life expectancy reached roughly 70 years by 1960 and has increased by approximately 0.2 years every year since (White, 2002). The decreased death rates among older Americans is attributed to factors such as improved access to health care, advances in medicine, healthier lifestyles, and better health before age 65 (National Center for Health Statistics, 2009). Over the approaching decades, the population will consist of more elderly than young people for the first time ever in known history (MacArthur Foundation Research Network on Aging, 2009). Currently, the number of Americans age 65 and older is projected to double by the year 2030 (Goldman et al., 2005).

Current evidence indicates that disability is declining among the elderly over time. This means the elderly have the possibility to enjoy a better quality of life, engage in more activities, and work into later ages. Disability is also very closely tied to medical spending, and its decline could potentially reduce public and private medical costs (Cutler, 2001). However, since the 1980s, researchers and policymakers have expressed concern that increased longevity will contribute not only to a larger elderly population but also to increased disability among this group (Goldman et al., 2005; Spillman, 2004). Moreover, the past decades have witnessed an increase in obesity and diabetes among young people, and the disability rates for this population have risen across all demographic and economic groups (Mokdad, Ford, et al., 2000; Mokdad, Serdula, et al., 2000). Health-care services are in greater demand to meet the needs of the growing disability rates (Buntin et al., 2004).

In terms of cost, current trends suggest that disability in the elderly is actually decreasing, but the utilization of institutional care—the most expensive type of long-term care—has remained static, signifying the decline in disability may not necessarily result in the decline of costs (Spillman, 2004). Some research shows that health expenditures for healthy elderly persons were similar to those for less healthy persons, even though the healthy individuals experienced greater longevity (Lubitz, Cai, Kramarow, & Lentzner, 2003). So, as healthy individuals live longer, the actual health-care costs over time may end up being about the same as the costs for their less healthy counterparts.

U.S. spending on health care has outpaced the gross domestic product by 3.5%-4.0% per year in recent decades, and the number of elderly is growing about 1.0% faster than the rest of the population (Fuchs, 1999). Many elderly individuals rely on Medicare and Social Security to assist in covering health costs and there is concern that these funds will be spread even thinner than they already are. Currently, on average, Medicare pays for less than half of the health care for the elderly, and Social Security benefits only provide less than half of the total income of individuals after the age of 65 (Fuchs, 1999). The crisis surrounding Medicare and Social Security does not have an easy fix, and some believe it will likely necessitate an overhaul of America's infrastructure.

Medicare and Social Security are key issues in the discussion about the welfare of aging Americans. Other issues of great importance may be overlooked by policymakers in their efforts to fix them. Many of the core institutions and structures in the United States are not prepared for the population shift and its subsequent effects. Factors, such as workforce participation, retirement, family, housing, and communities, will also need to be addressed to accommodate the growing numbers of aging adults (MacArthur Foundation Research Network on Aging, 2009; Maestas & Zissimopoulos, 2010).

The aging population is not a homogenous group. It is a mix of ethnicity, gender, socioeconomic status, culture, education, and geography. Some particular risk factors become more acute as individuals age. For example, older Americans are disproportionately likely to die by suicide. In addition, socioeconomic disparities in health are at their peak between the ages of 55 and 74 years old (Herd, 2006; House et al., 1990). Individuals living on a lower income, whether covered by Medicare or private insurance, are less likely to have the ability to pay the cost of deductibles, co-insurance, and procedures that are not covered. Moreover, a disparate number of Black Americans are in this income category, and data suggests that they often forgo procedures needed to improve their health (Eichner & Vladeck, 2005; Field & Jette, 2007). Unfortunately, even with comparable insurance coverage, Black Americans are more likely than White Americans to receive inferior health care (Geiger, 2006; Institute of Medicine, 2002). With the exception of some age and gender sub-groups within American Indians/Alaskan Natives, older Black Americans experience the highest rates of disability and limitations in the ability to engage in regular activities of any racial/ethnic group in its later years of life in the United States (Fuller-Thomson, Nuru-Jeter, Minkler, & Guralnik, 2009; Hummer, Benjamins, & Rogers, 2004).

Historically, women have lived longer than men in almost every country in the world (Austad, 2006). On average globally, women live approximately 5 years longer than men (United Nations, 2009). Today, a woman has a good chance of living into her 80s. And those who live to be 85 years old have a very good chance of living another 6 years (Newman & Brach, 2001). In addition, women continue to have a longer life expectancy and outnumber men at the age of 100 years 4 to 1 (Kannisto, 1994, 1996; Wilmoth & Lundstrom, 1996). Women do not live longer than men due to aging more slowly but because women are more robust at all ages (Austad, 2006). In virtually all age groups, males die at an earlier age than women in respect to practically all causes of death, including accidents, cancer, heart disease, flu, pneumonia, cerebrovascular accidents, and chronic obstructive pulmonary diseases (Austad, 2006; CDC, 1999; Kramarow, Lentzner, Rooks, Weeks, & Saydah, 1999). Men and the elderly are more likely to have fatal suicide attempts than are women and youth (CDC, 1999). Although suicide rates among older men are declining, older White men are three times as likely as older Black men and more than twice as likely as older Hispanic men to die from suicide. Moreover, suicide rates among older men tend to increase with age (National Center for Health Statistics, n.d.).

Paradoxically, men appear to experience less disability in later years compared to women (Austad, 2006; Newman & Brach, 2001). Women experience an increased rate of disability and higher rates of physical complaints, anxiety, and depression, reaching a peak in middle age and then dropping during post-menopause (Austad,

2006; Burt & Hendrick, 2005). Women have a tendency to suffer from non-terminal illnesses that have a negative impact on daily functioning (von Strauss, Agüero-Torres, Kåreholt, Winblad, & Fratiglioni, 2003). They also tend to have a higher risk for falls, accidents, and reduced physical and functional ability, and they have a higher rate of dependency on psychotropic drugs, benzodiazepines in particular (Austad, 2006; Simoni-Wastila, 2000). In addition, just the fact that women live longer results in more aging-related health issues and negative life events, such as losing loved ones and becoming widowed (Arber, Davidson, & Ginn, 2003; Perrig-Chiello & Hutchison, 2010).

Eldercare

Many individuals and families are faced with making choices on residential care for aging parents, spouses, partners, and loved ones. According to the U.S. Department of Health and Human Services (HHS), 1% of the American population aged 65-74 is in assisted living facilities (2004). The National Center for Assisted Living (2010) defines an assisted living facility (ALF) as "a congregate residential setting that provides or coordinates personal care services, 24-hour supervision, assistance (scheduled and unscheduled), activities, and health-related services," and it is designed to "minimize the need to move from the care setting," "accommodate individual residents' changing needs and preferences," "maximize residents' dignity, autonomy, privacy, independence, choice, and safety," and "encourage family and community involvement" (p. ix). ALFs are an option for many individuals and their loved ones due to the emphasis on "resident choice, dignity, and privacy" (National Center for Assisted Living, 2010, Introduction). To meet the growing demand for hospice and palliative care, these care options are increasingly more available to residents in assisted living situations (Cartwright, Miller, & Volpin, 2009). Although ALFs were originally designed for individuals with stable and predictable conditions, they are experiencing a transition as residents are increasingly older, experience more impaired functionality, and require more care than traditional ALFs (Ball et al., 2004).

In response to concern for the greater expenditures needed by the influx of aging individuals, programs have been developed to shift the focus from long-term assisted living to long-term community-based care (Kaye, LaPlante, & Harrington, 2009). Many individuals would make the choice to utilize community-based services as opposed to ALFs. A number of states have implemented federal programs, such as the Money Follows the Person (MFP) Rebalancing Demonstration Program (Deficit Reduction Act of 2005) in addition to state-initiated programs to facilitate transitions from nursing homes to the community (Kasper & O'Malley, 2006). Many elderly are admitted into nursing homes to rehabilitate and/or recover from an illness and then return to the community or stay in the facility to pass away (Arling, Kane, Cooke, & Lewis, 2010). A relatively small proportion of individuals stay in nursing homes for months or years at a time (Gill, Gahbauer, Han, & Allore, 2009; Jones, 2002; Kasper, 2005; Reschovsky, 1998). A move into a nursing home can result in a disconnection from the community and a subsequent loss of supportive resources like housing and friends. The longer an individual remains in assisted living, the less likely the individual will be able to transition into the community (Chapin, Baca, Macmillan, Rachlin, & Zimmerman, 2009; Coughlin, McBride, & Liu, 1990; Mehdizadeh, 2002) as community resources may decrease in availability (Kasper & O'Malley, 2006). In fact, less than 6% of Medicaid-eligible persons in nursing homes who remain there for 6 months or more actually transition back into their community each year (Wenzlow & Lipson, 2009).

A longstanding notion that families "abandon" their older relatives in nursing homes and forget about them is not always the case. Multiple studies indicate that family members do continue to visit and contribute to the care of their relatives after placing them in a nursing home. In recent decades, it has become more common for families to be incorporated into the daily lives of those in nursing homes. Families are seen less and less as "visitors" and more as an integral asset to the care of the elderly (Whitaker, 2009).

Elder abuse is a concern in institutional and home settings. As the population of older adults swells, the potential for instances of elder abuse increases. Elder abuse is defined as "a single or repeated act, or lack of appropriate action, occurring within any relationship where there is an expectation of trust which causes harm or distress to an older person" (Wolf, Daichman, & Bennett, 2002, p. 126). Abuse may come in the form of physical injury, physical illness, psychological distress, and financial ruin (Post et al., 2010). Studies have been conducted in multiple countries suggesting that 4%-6% of older adults experience some form of mistreatment (Comijs, Pot, Smit, Bouter, & Jonker, 1998; Kivela, Kongas-Saviaro, Kesti, Pahkala, & Ijas, 1992; Ogg & Bennett, 1992; Podnieks, 1992). Individuals in a long-term care facility are at considerable risk due to many of the limitations inherent in institutional settings, such as understaffing and lack of economic resources (Coyne, Reichman, & Berbig 1993; Post, Fulk, & Birosack 2008). The quality of nursing home care has been a long-standing concern. The issue gained wider media attention when the Institute of Medicine Committee on Nursing Home Regulation (1986) unearthed disturbing findings in the *Improving the Quality of Care in Nursing Homes Report*. Federal regulations were subsequently created to closely monitor and improve nursing homes' care of residents.

Biology and Physiology

Extensive strides have been made in understanding aging; however, it is still not clear what mechanism actually makes humans expire from old age. Aging is most often associated with the progressive loss of certain functions, the decrease of fertility, and the eventual death of the body. However, considering the process of aging from an evolutionary perspective, it would seem that aging is counter to the human instincts of survival and procreation. Aging cannot be explained by the "wear and tear" of living and raises many questions about why people age (Austad, 1997; Kirkwood, 1999;

Kirkwood & Austad, 2000; Kirkwood & Cremer, 1982; Rose, 1991). Many different theories surround the issue of aging and this section will touch on some of the most recent and salient information available.

Some evolutionary theories attempt to explain the phenomenon of aging; however, one agreed upon method of explaining aging does not exist. An early evolutionary theory proposed that aging is actually programmed into human bodies to limit the population size or speed up the turnover of generations so that people could adapt to changing environments. However, studies of other species in the wild show that aging rarely contributes to death. Most deaths in the wild affect the young and occur from outside factors such as predators and environmental factors. Most wild animals do not live long enough to experience the effects of aging (Kirkwood & Austad, 2000). Natural selection does not have time to actually assert direct influence on the process of aging. In species that do experience the effects of aging and in which aging contributes to death, it is unlikely that any of the aging genes would actually be beneficial to survival or procreation. And those that did not have any activated "aging genes" would be selected over individuals that had the genes (Kirkwood & Austad, 2000). According to the mutation accumulation theory, since death is usually caused by external factors and most species die young, the impact of natural selection weakens as aging occurs. Mutations of genes contribute to the aging process and go unchecked over generations (Charlesworth, 1994; Medawar, 1952). The theory of pleiotropy (a.k.a. antagonistic pleiotropy) posits that genes contributing to positive effects at an early age would be favored by natural selection even if they had negative effects at later ages (Williams, 1957). The disposable soma theory is based on the idea that metabolic resources will be utilized for the most productive time of life. Therefore, energy is used for reproduction and maintaining the body at earlier ages even at the cost of eventual aging and death (Kirkwood, 1977, 1996).

Interestingly, most individuals die of diseases that "have been largely unaffected by modern medicine or changes in the environment" (Juckett, 2010, p. xx). Modern medicine has increased the median lifespan, reduced rates of illness, and has enhanced the quality of life for those that do experience illness (Kort, Paneth, & Woude, 2009). However, individuals continue to die of age-related illnesses, and understanding of these illnesses is still in the nascent stages. There have been promising findings toward understanding the biological contributors to age-related illness and someday having a complete picture of what causes these illnesses (Juckett, 2010).

The discussion of aging raises questions about whether or not living a healthy lifestyle results in longevity and less illness (U.S. Department of Health and Human Services [HHS], 1990). The theory of compression of morbidity argues that practicing healthy lifestyles and other preventive practices will decrease disease and disability in older ages but only increase the lifespan marginally. The theory proposes that the cumulative effect of prevention efforts and healthy lifestyles is the reduction and compression of the amount of disease and disability experienced later in life into a shorter period (Hubert, Bloch, Oehlert, & Fries, 2002).

The process of *cellular senescence* may also help explain aging because it appears to play a causal role (Burton, Allen, Bird, & Faragher, 2007). Cellular senescence occurs when mitotic cells stop dividing and creating new cells. Most mitotic cells are in *quiescence*, an arrested state in which the cells stay dormant until being stimulated to proliferate, usually for the purpose of replacing other cells that have died (Burton, 2009). Mitotic tissues consist of these cells that have the ability to divide when stimulated. Senescent cells that can no longer proliferate to replace other cells begin to accumulate and affect the functioning of the tissue in which they reside. The accumulation of senescent cells also negatively affects other nearby cells. The senescent cells are no longer like other cells, and as they gradually accumulate, they begin to impair tissue function and predispose tissues to disease development and/or disease progression (Burton, 2009; Burton, Allen, Bird, & Faragher, 2005; Campisi, 1997a, 1997b; Burton et al., 2007).

One of the emerging major health threats of the 21st century is the cognitive decline that accompanies the aging process (Bishop, Lu, & Yankner, 2010). As life expectancy has increased, so has the prevalence of cognitive decline and dementia, mostly in the form of Alzheimer's disease, which affects almost 50% of U.S. adults over the age of 85 years old (Hebert, Scherr, Bienias, Bennett, & Evans, 2003). Cognitive decline is recognized in advanced aging even when there is no disease present. Some theories propose that the normal aging process results in the loss of white matter in the brain or the loss of the protective sheath around the nerves. Consequently, the properties of brain systems may change, or there may be a subtle disconnection between the regions of the brain that would normally work together (Head et al., 2004; O'Sullivan et al., 2001; Pfefferbaum et al., 2000, 2005; Salat et al., 2005). Studies have been limited, as many aspects of brain and physiological functioning have been difficult to measure (Andrews-Hanna et al., 2007).

Fortunately, within the past 15 years, more and more knowledge has been gained about the basic molecular mechanisms of aging. Studies suggest that the rate of aging and cognitive decline may actually be open to modification and not fixed (Bishop et al., 2010). Functional imaging studies reveal that when individuals age, less coordination exists between the different brain regions that serve the higher order cognitive functions. This reduced coordination is associated with poor performance in many cognitive areas (Andrews-Hanna et al., 2007). Brain activity also becomes less localized in some regions of the brain, which is believed to be a compensatory response to the natural aging process. Older individuals with less localized brain activity actually show better cognitive performance than older individuals who exhibit more localized brain activity (Cabeza, 2002; Cabeza, Anderson, Locantore, & McIntosh, 2002; Park & Reuter-Lorenz, 2009). As different parts of the brain become less active and functional due to the process of aging, many utilize other parts of the brain to compensate for the loss. These studies indicate that human brains are affected by age even in the absence of disease and that the potential capability to make up for the losses exists.

Prevention and Treatment

Unfortunately, no drug has been created yet that specifically targets senescent cells to help reign in the aging process. However, drugs are currently being developed to target specific cancer cells (Gillies & Fréchet, 2005) that could perhaps one day be adapted to target senescent cells (Burton, 2009). One promising type of intervention to aid in arresting the aging process and the associated diseases is *caloric restriction* (*CR*). CR is based on the notion that the lowered energy expended by cells during this type of intervention reduces the oxidation process that leads to cell death and subsequent disease and aging. CR involves mitochondria, which are the main source of cellular energy and are central to cellular processes (Cadenas & Davies, 2000). Mitochondria are also the main source of reactive oxygen species (ROS). ROS are generated by mitochondria or from other sites within or outside the cell and can cause damage to parts of the mitochondria and trigger the processes of cell death (Cadenas & Davies, 2000). Therefore, reducing metabolic rate by using CR may reduce oxygen consumption, which could decrease the creation of ROS and potentially increase lifespan (Heilbronn & Ravussin, 2003).

However, for some individuals, restricting food intake may be an extreme response to aging. But at the moment, not much else is under discussion when it comes to slowing down the inevitable course of action human bodies take. CR has been investigated for more than 70 years and provides the only intervention tested to date on mammals (mostly mice and rats) and other species (fish, flies, worms, and yeast) that repeatedly and strongly increases maximum life span while slowing down age-associated changes in the body (Heilbronn & Ravussin, 2003; Hursting, Lavigne, Berrigan, Perkins, & Barrett, 2003; Weindruch, 1996).

Death and Dying

Sociocultural Influences

Nineteenth-century Americans experienced death in a very different way than those living in the 21st century. The 19th century was wrought with death caused by infectious diseases, such as tuberculosis, diphtheria, scarlet fever, whooping cough, intestinal disorders, measles, smallpox, and malaria. In fact, most American cities faced these diseases in endemic and often epidemic proportions (Lundgren & Houseman, 2010). Death rates continued to rise until the late 19th and early 20th century, and then a noticeable decline occurred. It is difficult to pinpoint one particular factor that contributed to this decline because many factors influenced this trend. For instance, Americans had begun benefitting from the improvements brought about by the industrial revolution, which promoted better health through improved diet, housing, and personal hygiene (Leavitt & Numbers, 1985). Public health infrastructure had been created to improve sewer systems, water quality, and provide local boards of health. Medical care had improved and began to enjoy widely publicized accomplishments and greater trust from the public (Lundgren & Houseman, 2010).

Throughout the 19th century, most Americans died at home, but, as the century progressed, dying became more and more relegated to the institutional care of hospitals. In 1800, there were only two institutions in the United States that could reasonably be called hospitals (Rosenberg, 1987). The first hospital survey taken in 1873 identified 178 hospitals in existence, including mental hospitals (Reverby, 1987), and by 1909 there were 4,359 hospitals identified, exclusive of mental or chronic-disease hospitals (Rosenberg, 1987). The idea of caring for the dying at home went by the wayside and more sterile and detached methods of dealing with death became the norm. Death became shameful and burdensome, and the dying were consigned to isolation and institutional care as opposed to home care by family, neighbors, and friends. Some argue that the evolution of institutionalized care brought on the advent of death and dying being removed from everyday awareness and that it has influenced the American cultural stance on death and dying issues ever since. The argument contends that the normalcy and inevitability of death was replaced with an investment in the belief that medical science could "cure" death. If death was due to natural causes and if nature could be controlled, then it was a short leap to assume that death was the sign of failed medicine, no longer subjected to the whims of the natural world. Moreover, as infectious diseases were being eradicated due to medical advancements, it is not difficult to understand that faith would grow in the new scientific ideas to "treat" death (Lundgren & Houseman, 2010).

In addition, institutionalizing death and dying created businesses that ensured the distancing of a part of life that had traditionally been dealt with in the home. The profession of funeral directors began to gain status and create a specialized set of skills to meet the burgeoning need to move death out of the home setting. As the century progressed, cemeteries were moved farther out of the more densely inhabited areas into more rural and bucolic settings. The middle class in most American cities began to bury their dead in nicely landscaped, park-like settings away from the bustle of urban life. The business of cemeteries and funeral parlors became legitimized and integral to how death is currently perceived and managed (Lundgren & Houseman, 2010).

Aging not only brings individuals closer to their own death but also to the death of others around them at a gradually higher rate (Rook, 2000). This does not necessarily mean that the aged have to become more socially isolated. In fact, as people live into their later years, they may find a social network composed of others in similar positions, such as having lost a spouse or significant other (Ferraro, Mutran, & Barresi, 1984). An overview of current and past research identifies extensive variability regarding the issue of aging and increased loss of social and family supports. Some research shows that many older individuals thrive and strengthen social supports after the loss of a spouse or significant other. Other research indicates that certain factors increase the probability an individual will experience isolation and discontent in later years as family and social networks diminish (Cornwell, Laumann, & Schumm, 2008). For instance, a general myth about aging is that widows tend to be more resilient than widowers. Women have historically and more commonly been associated with being in charge of social contacts and being more capable of keeping a household together. However, their achievement of this is not always the case. Older men actually tend to find other partners much easier than older women and do not necessarily experience a greater loss of social connectedness in the face of the death of loved ones. Other factors such as personality and geography make a difference in the amount of isolation an aging individual experiences (Cornwell et al., 2008; LaLive d'Epinay, Cavalli, & Guillet, 2009-2010).

The majority of research reveals increased mental and physical well-being in those aging individuals given the opportunity to give their time and efforts to loved ones and others in need. Increased wellness also is exhibited in aging individuals that participate in social networks, such as church, community centers, volunteering, family, friends, neighbors, and any interests that give meaning to their lives and help them cope with the effects of death (Cornwell et al., 2008; Krause, Herzog, & Baker, 1992; LaLive d'Epinay et al., 2009-2010; Thomas, 2010). Providing opportunities for the elderly to be contributing members of their families and communities may not only increase positive health outcomes for the aging but change the general perception of aging to a time of productivity instead of decline.

End-of-Life Care
End-of-life care has become a much discussed topic in the last couple of decades due to the growing aging population, increase in lingering chronic illnesses, and improved but controversial life support technology (Gruneir et al., 2007). End-of-life care encompasses both hospice and palliative care services. It also addresses the paradox of most Americans preferring a home death but the majority of them dying in institutional settings, such as hospitals or nursing homes (Hays, Galanos, Palmer, McQuoid, &

Flint, 2001; Tang, 2003). Institutions, such as assisted living facilities, are evolving and modifying services to create environments that are more reminiscent of a home setting and are often preferred by individuals facing life-threatening situations.

Philosophically, end-of-life care issues revolve around the rights of individuals to make the most appropriate choice to fit their idea of a "good death." Reports and large-scale research projects have highlighted the nature of the end-of-life controversies and how to improve the services in demand by individuals facing death (Aulino & Foley, 2001; Field & Cassel, 1997; Foley & Gelband, 2001; SUPPORT principal investigators, 1995). As the debates continue, end-of-life care advocates are making progress in assuring that the needs of Americans are being met.

Hospice services in America began with the Connecticut Hospice in March 1974. Today there are over 2,884 Medicare-certified hospice programs and an additional 200 volunteer hospices with approximately 1.5 million Americans utilizing hospice treatment in recent years (Icanberry, n.d.). The hospice movement in the US is committed to helping people die "well" with an emphasis on providing the majority of care at home or homelike settings. The hospice concept is derived from medieval times and symbolizes a place where "travelers, pilgrims, and the sick, wounded or dying could find rest and comfort" ("Hospice," n.d.). The contemporary hospice movement offers a program of care for patients and families who are facing a life-threatening illness. It is not a particular place of care but more of a concept of care emphasizing the comfort of ailing individuals rather than trying to cure them. The focus is on quality of life as opposed to quantity. Hospice provides medical, emotional, spiritual, and practical support to the dying and their family. Hospice offers services to those who have a limited life expectancy and have made a decision to spend their last days at home or in a homelike setting ("Hospice," n.d.). However, the proportion of deaths where hospice is involved remains small (Weitzen, Teno, Fennell, & Mor, 2003).

The difference between hospice care and palliative care is that palliative care addresses the needs of individuals with life-threatening illnesses at any point, regardless of life expectancy, and hospice provides care for those who can no longer benefit from standard medical care and are in the last stages of terminal illness (Icanberry, n.d.). In terms of insurance coverage, Medicare/Medicaid, most private insurance plans, HMOs, and other managed care providers cover hospice services, but palliative care is not as commonly covered. Some private insurance companies may cover palliative care, and it is imperative for consumers to ask how these services will actually be covered and how much they will be responsible to pay (Icanberry, n.d.).

Despite the palliative and hospice care movements advocating for end-of-life care rights, many barriers still exist in terms of access to quality end-of-life care services, including systemic factors, such as the emphasis on curative and life-sustaining interventions as opposed to supportive care, health-care financing and service delivery infrastructures that promote decreased continuity of care, a lack of trained service providers, and a lack of evidence-based research in the area (Emanuel, von Gunten, & Ferris, 2000; Field & Cassel, 1997; Morrison, 2005). Other issues act as barriers, including the unpredictable nature of terminal illnesses, difficulties that arise between familial and social relationships, and the inevitable complex-care needs required for a dying individual and their loved ones (Kramer & Auer, 2005). Furthermore, hospice and palliative care are typically underutilized and oftentimes inaccessible to the poor, racial and ethnic minorities, and elders who are isolated or suffer from unknown ailments (Gardner & Kramer, 2009-2010). Some states have recently, even in spite of economic downturns, increased aid to needy individuals that typically would be unable to afford an assisted living facility (National Center for Assisted Living, 2010).

Although continued findings indicate that Americans prefer to die at home, most of the deaths in the United States occur in an institutional setting, the acute-care hospital being the number one site of death for those with chronic illnesses. However, from the late-1980s to 2001, the number of home deaths increased from 16% to 23%. A noteworthy aspect is the differences between some locations. Oregon reports a high of 38.4% of its residents' deaths as home deaths whereas Washington, DC registers a low of 12.4% of its deaths as home deaths (Brown University Center for Gerontology and Healthcare Research, 2009). There are also differences between certain racial/ethnic groups. For example, African Americans and Latino/Hispanic populations have a greater likelihood of dying in a hospital setting than at home (Gruneir et al., 2007).

The Institute of Medicine defines a "good death" as one with minimal suffering that satisfies the wishes of dying patients and their families while adhering to current medical, cultural, and ethical standards (Field & Cassel, 1997). A growing amount of research indicates that most individuals coping with life-threatening illnesses wish to be free of pain and symptoms (Heyland et al., 2006; Vig & Pearlman, 2004), to be treated with dignity and respect (Chochinov et al., 2002; Steinhauser et al., 2000), and to maintain a sense of autonomy and control over their last days (McSkimming et al., 1999; Vig & Pearlman, 2004; Singer, Martin, & Kellner, 1999). People reported that they prefer to be completely informed about their diagnosis and be given time to put their affairs in order (Heyland et al., 2006; McCormick & Conley, 1995; Terry, Olson, Wilss, & Boulton-Lewis, 2006) and not be a burden to their loved ones (McPherson, Wilson, & Murray, 2007; Vig & Pearlman, 2004). Typically, individuals stated that they would not approve and do not desire the use of artificial supports to sustain their life if death is imminent (Heyland et al., 2006; Singer et al., 1999). The idea of a "good death" is in many ways based on individual preferences and is something that the majority of Americans believe is an important issue (National Center for Assisted Living, 2010).

We interviewed Margaret, a 73-year-old woman, requesting her thoughts on aging, death, and dying. For Margaret, it is vital to begin each morning by saying "Girl, you're going to have a good day today." This ritual began when she had been very depressed after her husband's death. Work had helped Margaret with his physical absence, but her conviction for telling herself she was going to have a good day and then making an effort to do so was crucial to her positive mindset and alleviating her depression. Margaret believes her husband still lives and exists with her in their home but that she just cannot touch him. And because of his presence in their home, she will not move from it until she has also passed away.

Margaret does not allow herself to grow old, to see herself as old or bitter and quit living. She will not dye her hair because she believes she has earned every single one of her gray hairs and that they do not look bad. In fact, she wishes her hair was all gray, but she does not think it will happen because she is having fun and enjoying life. Until her recent retirement, her kids would constantly ask her why she didn't retire. She would tell them that she wasn't ready and that she just didn't want to stop working. After Margaret celebrated her 70th birthday, she decided it was time she did do things for herself.

Margaret's many activities keep her young. She avidly plays Mah Jongg and Trivial Pursuit. She also enjoys painting and weaving. She keeps some company with young people, but not necessarily because they make her feel young. Margaret believes they, like her, just don't let themselves get old, and that is what she enjoys about the people she chooses to be around. Some activities are more difficult for her these days, but she has replaced them with others. Margaret once kept a daily walking route and danced frequently. Now, she does other exercises everyday. She has also decided to eat healthier and has lost weight as a result.

Recently, Margaret explicitly told her daughter that if she was ever to become unable to take care of herself, she would not wish for her daughter or her other kids to tend to her. Margaret has made arrangements for that to be carried out. The philosophy that Margaret lives by and would promote among her fellow retirees would be to not allow for idleness and for everyone to be active. She does not want to get Alzheimer's disease because she was lax.

Margaret has no desire to cease living now, but she does not fear death. Margaret believes she knows where she will go after death, and to her understanding, it is not a bad place.

An outlook on aging, death, and dying was gathered from Susan, a 60-year-old woman. Susan's account of her experience with aging, death, and dying begins when she was young. She was in a rush toward adulthood then because she believed being an adult meant freedom to make her own decisions. As a young adult, Susan realized the nurturing and security of her childhood had gone, but a future in the real world and its wide array of life experiences enthralled her. At that time, old age seemed so distant.

Now, Susan reflects on her career, marriage, and family. She takes pleasure in being a wise grandparent and meditating on her memories. Susan recognizes she has more wrinkles and aches, and she worries more about the future, how her body will endure and how much time and productivity she has left. Susan believes everything lost with age is replaced by other good things. She notices her priorities have changed with age and she has learned to compromise. She has accepted how her life has changed in both good ways and bad. And that death is inevitable. But she will not tolerate becoming a burden to her loved ones. Susan wants to be ready if something should happen to her. She wants her assets to be organized for easy final arrangements, and she plans to dispose of every unnecessary possession. She has also prepared a living will (advance directive). She hopes that, when the time comes, she will not suffer and face it bravely. At the end of her life, Susan wishes to feel content with accomplishments that were beneficial to others.

Along with living a full life and just doing the best she can with no regrets, another challenge she faces is staying healthy. To others, Susan suggests not being afraid of aging or death and dying. She also recommends using moisturizers. Humor is a great coping mechanism for her. Acceptance of herself and her life's work and acceptance of the inevitability of aging and dying has given Susan an enduring positive outlook.

Conclusion

The issue of aging, death, and dying is one that affects every individual. As medical science continues to pursue methods to stave off aging and death, people benefit by living longer and healthier. The majority of infectious diseases have been eradicated in the industrialized parts of the world and strides are being made in understanding how to deal with the threat of chronic illnesses. As individuals live longer, the culture of aging and death is being redefined, as can be seen in the hospice and palliative-care movement and the increased attention toward nursing care. Unfortunately, the disadvantaged and disenfranchised continue to experience disparities in this care. Individuals are left behind, unable to access the resources available to other sectors of society. Inevitably, addressing these issues is rising to the forefront as medical science progresses and the culture of aging and dying evolves to give people more options and advantages.

Recommendations

Although it may be impossible to eradicate the aging process and eventual death, many lifestyle choices can mediate the deterioration associated with growing older. Engaging in healthful behaviors, such as exercise and leisure activities, regulating sleep and nutrition, and regular doctor visits, can contribute to an increased quality of life and lessen the impact of the aging process. It is also important to maintain mental health and to exercise the mind regularly to manage the effects of aging on the brain. Staying informed regarding current health issues related to aging, death, and dying is key to understanding what to expect from the process and being empowered to cope with death. In addition, planning for a "good death" is increasingly warranted as end-of-life care resources are expanding to give more choices to Americans, such as home-based palliative and hospice care. Acknowledging the fact that death is part of the normal life cycle can give one time to consider the options and choose the resources that are most appropriate for the pursuit of a "good death." Aging and death are inevitable, but fortunately, knowledge is growing in this area and ample information is available to help people enjoy their later years and die in a manner that is most comfortable and agreeable to them.

Selected Resources

Administration on Aging
One Massachusetts Avenue, NW
Washington, DC 20001
Office of the Assistant Secretary for Aging: 202-401-4634; Public Inquiries: 202-619-0724
Eldercare Locator (to find local resources): 800-677-1116; Fax: 202-357-3555
aoainfo@aoa.hhs.gov
www.aoa.gov/

American Psychological Association
750 First Street, NE
Washington, DC 20002-4242
800-374-2721; 202-336-5500; TDD/TTY: 202-336-6123
www.apa.org/topics/death/index.aspx

Centers for Disease Control and Prevention (CDC)
Healthy Aging Program
4770 Buford Highway, NE, Mailstop K-45
Atlanta, GA 30341-3717
800-CDC-INFO (800-232-4636); TTY: 888-232-6348
www.cdc.gov/aging/

Hospicenet.org
401 Bowling Avenue, Suite 51
Nashville, TN 37205-5124
info@hospicenet.org
www.hospicenet.org/

MedlinePlus
U.S. National Library of Medicine
8600 Rockville Pike
Bethesda, MD 20894
www.nlm.nih.gov/medlineplus/endoflifeissues.html

National Institute on Aging
Building 31, Room 5C27
31 Center Drive, MSC 2292
Bethesda, MD 20892
www.nia.nih.gov/

References

Andrews-Hanna, J. R., Snyder, A. Z., Vincent, J. L., Lustig, C., Head, D., Raichle, M. E., & Buckner, R. L. (2007). Disruption of large-scale brain systems in advanced aging. *Neuron, 56*(5), 924-935.

Arber, S., Davidson, K., & Ginn, J. (2003). *Gender and ageing, changing roles and relationships.* Philadelphia, PA: Open University Press.

Arling, G., Kane, R. L., Cooke, V., & Lewis, T. (2010, June). Targeting residents for transitions from nursing home to community. *Health Services Research, 45*(3), 691-711.

Aulino, F., & Foley, K. (2001). The project on death in America. *Journal of the Royal Society of Medicine, 94*(9), 492-495.

Austad, S. N. (1997). *Why we age.* New York, NY: Wiley.

Austad, S. N. (2006). Why women live longer than men: Sex differences in longevity. *Gender Medicine, 3*(2), 79-92.

Ball, M., Whittington, F., Perkins, M., Patterson, V., Hollingsworth, C., King, S. V., . . . Combs, B. L. (2004). Managing decline in assisted living: The key to aging in place. *Journal of Gerontology: Social Sciences, 59B*, S202-S212.

Bishop, N. A., Lu, T., & Yankner, B. A. (2010, March). Neural mechanisms of ageing and cognitive decline. *Nature, 464*, 529-535.

Brown University Center for Gerontology and Health Care Research. (2009). Facts on dying: Policy relevant data on care at the end of life. Retrieved September 25, 2010, from *http:// www.chcr.brown.edu/dying/factsondying.htm*

Buntin, M. J. B., Escarce, J. J., Goldman, D., Kan, H., Laugesen, M. J., & Shekelle, P. (2004). Increased Medicare expenditures for physicians' services: What are the causes? *Inquiry 41*(1), 83-94.

Burt, V. K., & Hendrick, V. C. (2005). *Clinical manual of women's mental health.* Arlington, VA: American Psychiatric Publishing.

Burton, D. G. A. (2009). Cellular senescence, ageing and disease. *Age, 31*(1), 1-9.

Burton, D. G. A., Allen, M. C., Bird, J. L. E., & Faragher, R. G. A. (2005). Bridging the gap: Ageing, pharmacokinetics and pharmacodynamics. *Journal of Pharmacy and Pharmacology, 57*(6), 671-679.

Burton, D. G. A., Sheerin, A., Ostler, E. L., Smith, K., Giles, P. J., Lowe, J., . . . Faragher, R. G. A. (2007). Cyclin D1 over-expression permits the reproducible detection of senescent human vascular smooth muscle cells. *Annals of the New York Academy of Sciences, 1119,* 20-31.

Cabeza, R. (2002). Hemispheric asymmetry reduction in older adults: The HAROLD model. *Psychology and Aging, 17*(1), 85-100.

Cabeza, R., Anderson, N. D., Locantore, J. K., & McIntosh, A. R. (2002). Aging gracefully: Compensatory brain activity in high-performance older adults. *NeuroImage, 17*(3), 1394-1402.

Cadenas, E., & and Davies, K. J. A. (2000). Mitochondrial free radical generation, oxidative stress, and aging. *Free Radical Biology & Medicine, 29*(3/4), 222-230,

Campisi, J. (1997a). Aging and cancer: The double-edged sword of replicative senescence. *Journal of the American Geriatric Society, 45*(4), 482-488.

Campisi, J. (1997b). The biology of replicative senescence. *European Journal of Cancer, 33*(5), 703-709.

Cartwright, J. C., Miller, L., & Volpin, M. (2009). Hospice in assisted living: Promoting good quality care at end of life. *Gerontologist, 49*(4), 508-516.

Centers for Disease Control and Prevention. (1999). Mortality patterns in the United States, 1997. *Morbidity and Mortality Weekly Report (MMWR), 282,* 664-668.

Chapin, R., Baca, B., Macmillan, K., Rachlin, R., & Zimmerman, M. (2009). Residential outcomes for nursing facility applicants who have been diverted: Where are they 5 years later? *Gerontologist, 49*(1), 46-56.

Charlesworth, B. (1994). *Evolution in age-structured populations.* Cambridge, England: Cambridge University Press.

Chochinov, H., Hack, T., Hassard, L., Kristjianson, S., McClement, S., & Harlos, M. (2002). Dignity in the terminally ill: A cross-sectional, cohort study. *The Lancet, 360*(9350), 2026-2030.

Comijs, H. C., Pot, A. M., Smit, J. H., Bouter L. M., Jonker, C. (1998). Elder abuse in the community: Prevalence and consequences. *Journal of the American Geriatrics Society, 46*(7), 885-888.

Cornwell, B., Laumann, E. O., Schumm, L. P. (2008, April). The social connectedness of older adults: A national profile. *American Sociological Review, 73*(2), 185.

Coughlin, T. A., McBride, T. D., & Liu, K. (1990). Determinants of transitory and permanent nursing home admissions. *Medical Care, 28*(7), 616-631.

Coyne, A. C., Reichman, W. E., & Berbig, L. J. (1993). The relationship between dementia and elder abuse. *The American Journal of Psychiatry, 150*, 643-646.

Cutler, D. M. (2001). The reduction in disability among the elderly. *Proceedings of the National Academy of Sciences (PNAS), 98*, 6546-6547.

Deficit Reduction Act of 2005, Pub. L. No. 109-171, § 6071, 120 Stat. 4 (2006).

Eichner, J., & Vladeck, B. C. (2005). Medicare as a catalyst for reducing health disparities. *Health Affairs, 24*, 365-375.

Emanuel, L., von Gunten, C., & Ferris, F. (2000). Gaps in end-of-life care. *Archives of Family Medicine, 9*, 1176-1180.

Ferraro, K. F., Mutran, E., & Barresi, C. M. (1984). Widowhood, health, and friendship support in later life. *Journal of Health and Social Behavior, 25*, 246-59.

Field, M. J., & Cassel, C. K. (Eds.). (1997). *Approaching death: Improving care at the end of life.* Washington, DC: National Academies Press.

Field, M. J., & Jette, A. M. (Eds.). (2007). *The future of disability in America.* Washington, DC: National Academies Press.

Foley, K. M., & Gelband, H. (Eds.). (2001). *Improving palliative care for cancer.* Washington, DC: National Academies Press.

Fried, L. P. (2000). Epidemiology of aging. *Epidemiologic Reviews, 22*(1), 95-106.

Fuchs, V. (1999). Provide, provide: The economics of aging. In A. Rattenmaier & T. R. Saving (Eds.), *Medicare reform: Issues and answers.* Chicago, IL: University of Chicago Press.

Fuller-Thomson, E., Nuru-Jeter, A., Minkler, M., & Guralnik, J. M. (2009, August). Black–White disparities in disability among older Americans further untangling the role of race and socioeconomic status. *Journal of Aging and Health, 21*(5), 677-698.

Gardner, D. S., & Kramer, B. J. (2009-2010). End-of-life concerns and care preferences: Congruence among terminally ill elders and their family caregivers. *Omega, 60*(3), 273-297.

Geiger, H. J. (2006). Health disparities: What do we know? What do we need to know? What should we know? In A. J. Schultz & L. Mullings (Eds.), *Gender, race, class and health* (pp. 261-288). San Francisco, CA: Jossey-Bass.

Gill, T. M., Gahbauer, E. A., Han, L., & Allore, H. G. (2009). Functional trajectories in older persons admitted to a nursing home with disability after an acute hospitalization. *Journal of American Geriatric Society, 57*(2), 195-201.

Gillies, E. R., & Fréchet, J. M. J. (2005). pH-responsive copolymer assemblies for controlled release of doxorubicin. *Bioconjugate Chemistry, 16*, 361-368.

Goldman, D. P., Baoping, S., Bhattacharya, J., Garber, A. M., Hurd, M. Joyce, G. F., . . . Shekelle, P. G. (2005). Consequences of health trends and medical innovation for the future elderly: When demographic trends temper the optimism of biomedical advances, how will tomorrow's elderly fare? [Web Exclusive]. *Health Affairs,* W5-R5–W5-R17.

Gruneir, A., Mor, V., Weitzen, S., Truchil, R., Teno, J., & Roy, J. (2007). Where people die: A multilevel approach to understanding influences on site of death in America. *Medical Care Research and Review, 64*(4), 351-378.

Hays, J. C., Galanos, A. N., Palmer, T. A., McQuoid, D. R., & Flint,

E. P. (2001). Preference for place of death in a continuing care retirement community. *Gerontologist, 41*(1), 123-128.

Head, D., Buckner, R. L., Shimony, J. S., Williams, L. E., Akbudak, E., Conturo, T. E., . . . Snyder, A. Z. (2004). Differential vulnerability of anterior white matter in nondemented aging with minimal acceleration in dementia of the Alzheimer type: Evidence from diffusion tensor imaging. *Cerebral Cortex, 14,* 410-423.

Hebert, L. E., Scherr, P. A., Bienias, J. L., Bennett, D. A., & Evans, D. A. (2003). Alzheimer disease in the U.S. population: Prevalence estimates using the 2000 census. *Archives of Neurology, 60*(8), 1119-1122.

Heilbronn, L. K., & Ravussin, E. (2003). Calorie restriction and aging: Review of the literature and implications for studies in humans. *American Journal of Clinical Nutrition, 78,* 361-369.

Herd, P. (2006). Do functional health inequalities decrease in old age? Educational status and functional decline among the 1931-1941 birth cohort. *Research on Aging, 28,* 375-392.

Heyland, D., Dodek, P., Rocker, G., Groll, D., Gafni, A., Pichora, D., . . . Lam, M. (2006). What matters most in end-of-life care: Perceptions of seriously ill patients and their family members. *Canadian Medical Association Journal, 174*(5), 627-633.

Hospice: The hospice concept. (n.d.). Retrieved September 23, 2010, from http://www.hospicenet.org/html/concept.html

House, J. S., Kessler, R. C., Herzog, A. R., Mero, R., Kinney, A. M., & Breslow, M. (1990). Age, socioeconomic status, and health. *Milbank Quarterly, 68,* 383-411.

Hubert, H. B., Bloch, D. A., Oehlert, J. W., & Fries, J. F. (2002).

Lifestyle habits and compression of morbidity. *Journal of Gerontology: Medical Sciences, 57A*(6), M347-M351.

Hummer, R., Benjamins, M., & Rogers, R. (2004). Race/ethnic disparities in health and mortality among the elderly: A documentation and examination of social factors. In N. Anderson, B. Bulatao, & B. Cohen (Eds.), *Critical perspectives on racial and ethnic differences in health in later life* (pp. 53-94). Washington, DC: National Research Council.

Hursting, S. D., Lavigne, J. A., Berrigan, D., Perkins, S. N., & Barrett, J. C. (2003). Calorie restriction, aging, and cancer prevention: Mechanisms of action and applicability to humans. *Annual Review of Medicine, 54*, 131-152.

Icanberry, A. (n.d.). What's the difference between hospice and palliative care? Retrieved September, 23 2010, from http://www. caring.com/articles/whats-the-difference-between-hospice-and-palliative-care

Institute of Medicine. (2002). *Unequal treatment: Confronting racial and ethnic disparities in health care.* Washington, DC: National Academies Press.

Institute of Medicine Committee on Nursing Home Regulation. (1986). *Improving the quality of care in nursing homes.* Washington, DC: National Academies Press.

Jones, A. (2002). The national nursing home survey: 1999 summary. *Vital and Health Statistics Series 13: Data from the National Health Survey, 13*(152), 1-116.

Juckett, D. A. (2010). What determines age-related disease: Do we know all the right questions? *Age, 32*(2), 155-160.

Kannisto, V. (1994). Development of oldest-old mortality, 1995-1990: Evidence from 28 developed countries. *Odense Monographs on*

Population Aging, Vol. 1. Odense, Denmark: Odense University Press.

Kannisto, V. (1996). The advancing frontier of survival. *Odense Monographs on Population Aging, Vol. 3.* Odense, Denmark: Odense University Press.

Kasper, J. (2005). *Who stays and who goes home: Using national data on nursing home discharges and long-stay residents to draw implications for nursing home transition programs.* Retrieved from http://www.kff.org/medicaid/upload/7386.pdf

Kasper, J., & O'Malley, M. (2006). *Nursing home transition programs: Perspectives of Medicaid care planners.* Retrieved from http://www.kff.org/medicaid/upload/7483.pdf

Kaye, H. S., LaPlante, M. P., & Harrington, C. (2009). Do non-institutional long-term care services reduce Medicaid spending? *Health Affairs, 28*(1), 262-272.

Kirkwood, T. B. L. (1977). Evolution of ageing. *Nature, 270,* 301-304.

Kirkwood, T. B. L. (1996). Human senescence. *BioEssays, 18,* 1009-1016.

Kirkwood, T. B. L. (1999). *Time of our lives: The science of human ageing.* New York, NY: Oxford University Press.

Kirkwood, T. B. L., & Austad, S. N. (2000, November). Why do we age? *Nature, 408,* 233-238.

Kirkwood, T. B. L., & Cremer, T. (1982). Cytogerontology since 1881: A reappraisal of August Weismann and a review of modern progress. *Human Genetics, 60*(2), 101-121.

Kivela, S. L., Kongas-Saviaro, P., Kesti, E., Pahkala, K., & Ijas, M.

L. (1992). Abuse in old age: Epidemiological data from Finland. *Journal of Elder Abuse and Neglect, 4*(3), 1-18.

Kort, E. J., Paneth, N., & Woude, G. F. V. (2009). The decline in U.S. cancer mortality in people born since 1925. *Cancer Research, 69*(16), 6500-6505.

Kramarow, E., Lentzner, H., Rooks, R., Weeks, J., & Saydah, S. (1999). *Health and aging chartbook. Health, United States, 1999.* Hyattsville, MD: National Center for Health Statistics.

Kramer, B. J., & Auer, C. (2005). Challenges to providing end-of-life care to low-income elders with advanced chronic disease: Lessons learned from a model program. *The Gerontologist, 45,* 651-660.

Krause, N., Herzog, A. R., & Baker, E. (1992). Providing support to others and well-being in later life. *Journal of Gerontology: Social Sciences, 47,* 300-311.

LaLive d'Epinay, C. J., Cavalli, S., & Guillet, L. A. (2009-2010). Bereavement in very old age: Impact on health and relationships of the loss of a spouse, child, a sibling, or a close friend. *Omega, 60*(4), 301-325.

Leavitt, J. W., & Numbers, R. L. (1985). *Sickness and health in America: Readings in the history of medicine and public health.* Madison, WI: University of Wisconsin Press.

Lubitz, J., Cai, L., Kramarow, E., & Lentzner, H. (2003). Health, life expectancy, and health care spending among the elderly. *New England Journal of Medicine, 349*(11), 1048-1055.

Lundgren, B., & Houseman, C. (2010). Banishing death: The disappearance of the appreciation of mortality. *Omega: Journal of Death & Dying, 61*(3), 223-249.

MacArthur Foundation Research Network on an Aging Society.

(2009, Fall). Facts and fictions about an aging America. *Contexts, 8*(4), 16-21.

Maddison, A. (2001). *The world economy: A millennial perspective.* Paris, France: OECD Development Centre.

Maestas, M., & Zissimopoulos, J. (2010, Winter). How longer work lives ease the crunch of population aging. *Journal of Economic Perspectives, 24*(1), 139-160.

McCormick, T., & Conley, B. (1995). Patients' perspectives on dying and on the care of dying patients. *Western Journal of Medicine, 163*(3), 236-243.

McPherson, C., Wilson, K., & Murray, M. (2007). Feeling like a burden: Exploring the perspectives of patients at the end of life. *Social Science & Medicine, 64*(2), 417-427.

McSkimming, S., Hodges, M., Super, A., Driever, M., Schoessler, M., Franey, S. G., & Lee, M. (1999). The experience of life-threatening illness: Patients' and their loved ones' perspectives. *Journal of Palliative Medicine, 2*(2), 173-184.

Medawar, P. B. (1952). *An unsolved problem of biology.* London, England: Lewis.

Mehdizadeh, S. A. (2002). Health and long-term care use trajectories of older disabled women. *Gerontologist, 42*(3), 304-314.

Mokdad, A. H., Ford, E. S., Bowman, B. A., Nelson, D. E., Engelgau, M. M., Vinicor, F., & Marks, J. S. (2000). Diabetes trends in the U.S.: 1990-1998. *Diabetes Care, 23*(9), 1278-1283.

Mokdad, A. H., Serdula, M. K., Dietz, W. H., Bowman, B. A., Marks, J. S., & Koplan, J. P. (2000). The continuing epidemic of obesity in the United States. *Journal of the American Medical Association, 284*(13), 1650-1651.

Morrison, S. (2005). Health care system factors affecting end-of-life care. *Journal of Palliative Medicine, 8*(Suppl. 1), S79-S87.

National Center for Assisted Living. (2010). *Assisted living state regulatory review 2010.* Retrieved on September 24, 2010, from http://www.ahcancal.org/ncal/resources/Pages/AssistedLivingRegulations.aspx

National Center for Health Statistics. (n.d.). Mortality by underlying and multiple cause, ages 18+: US, 1981–2006. Retrieved September 23, 2010, from Health Data Interactive website: www.cdc.gov/nchs/hdi.htm

National Center for Health Statistics. (2010). *Health, United States, 2009: With special feature on medical technology.* Hyattsville, MD: Author. Retrieved from http://www.cdc.gov/nchs/data/hus/hus09.pdf#105

Newman, A. B., & Brach, J. S. (2001). Gender gap in longevity and disability in older persons. *Epidemiological Reviews, 23*(2), 343-350.

Ogg, J., & Bennett, G. (1992). Elder abuse in Britain. *British Medical Journal, 305*(6860), 998-999.

O'Sullivan, M., Jones, D. K., Summers, P. E., Morris, R. G., Williams, S. C., & Markus, H. S. (2001). Evidence for cortical "disconnection" as a mechanism of age-related cognitive decline. *Neurology, 57*, 632-638.

Park, D. C., & Reuter-Lorenz, P. (2009). The adaptive brain: Aging and neurocognitive scaffolding. *Annual Review of Psychology, 60*, 173-196.

Perrig-Chiello, P., & Hutchison, S. (2010). Health and well-being in old age: The pertinence of a gender mainstreaming approach in research. *Gerontology, 56*(2), 208-213.

Pfefferbaum, A., Sullivan, E. V., Hedehus, M., Lim, K. O., Adalsteinsson, E., & Moseley, M. (2000). Age-related decline in brain white matter anisotropy measured with spatially corrected echo-planar diffusion tensor imaging. *Magnetic Resonance in Medicine, 44*, 259-268.

Pfefferbaum, A., Adalsteinsson, E., and Sullivan, E.V. (2005). Frontal circuitry degradation marks healthy adult aging: evidence from diffusion tensor imaging. *Neuroimage, 26*, 891–899.

Podnieks, E. (1992). National survey on abuse of the elderly in Canada. *Journal of Elder Abuse and Neglect, 4*, 5-58.

Post, L. A., Fulk, R., & Birosack, B. J. (2008). Violence prevention informatic systems. *The International Journal of Technology, Knowledge and Society, 4*, 155-62.

Post, L., Page, C., Conner, T., Prokhorov, A., Fang, Y., & Biroscak, B. J. (2010). Elder abuse long-term care: Types, patterns, and risk factors. *Research on Aging, 32*(3), 323-348.

Reschovsky, J. D. (1998). The demand for post-acute and chronic care in nursing homes. *Medical Care, 36*(4), 475-490.

Reverby, S. M. (1987). *Ordered to care: The dilemma of American nursing, 1850-1945.* New York, NY: Cambridge University Press.

Rook, K. S. (2000). The evolution of social relationships in later adulthood. In S. H. Qualls & N. Abeles (Eds.), *Psychology and the aging revolution. How we adapt to longer life* (pp. 173-191). Washington, DC: American Psychological Association.

Rose, M. R. (1991). *Evolutionary Biology of Ageing.* New York, NY: Oxford University Press.

Rosenberg, C. E. (1987). *The care of strangers: The rise of America's hospital system.* New York, NY: Basic Books.

Salat, D. H., Tuch, D. S., Greve, D. N., van der Kouwe, A. J., Hevelone, N. D., Zaleta, A.K., . . . Dale, A. M. (2005). Age-related alterations in white matter microstructure measured by diffusion tensor imaging. *Neurobiology* of *Aging, 26*, 1215-1227.

Simoni-Wastila, L. (2000). The use of abusable prescription drugs: The role of gender. *Journal of Women's Health and Gender-Based Medicine, 9*(3), 289-297.

Singer, P., Martin, D., & Kellner, M. (1999). Quality end-of-life care: Patients' perspectives. *Journal of the American Medical Association, 281*, 163-168.

Spillman, B. C. (2004). Changes in elderly disability rates and the implications for health care utilization and cost. *The Milbank Quarterly, 82*(1), 157-94.

Steinhauser, A., Christakis N., Clipp E., McNeilly, M., McIntyre, L., & Tulsky, J. (2000). Factors considered important at the end of life by patients, family, physicians, and other care providers. *Journal of the American Medical Association, 284*(19), 2476-2482.

SUPPORT principal investigators. (1995). A controlled trial to improve care for seriously ill hospitalized patients: The study to understand prognosis and preferences for outcomes and risks for treatments (SUPPORT). *Journal of the American Medical Association, 274*(20), 1591-1598.

Tang, S. T. (2003). Determinants of hospice home care use among terminally ill cancer patients. *Nursing Research, 52*, 217-225.

Terry, W., Olson, L., Wilss, L., & Boulton-Lewis, G. (2006). Experience of dying: Concerns of dying patients and of carers. *Internal Medicine Journal, 36*(6), 338-346.

Thomas, P.A. (2010). Is it better to give or to receive? Social support and the well-being of older adults. *Journal of Gerontology: Social Sciences, 65B*(3), 351-357.

United Nations, Department of Economic and Social Affairs, Population Division. (2009). *World population prospects: The 2008 revision*. New York, NY: Author.

U. S. Department of Health and Human Services. (1990). *Healthy people 2000: Health promotion and disease prevention objectives*. Washington, DC: Government Printing Office.

U.S. Department of Health and Human Services, National Center for Health Statistics. (2004).

National nursing home survey: Number and rates of current residents by selected characteristics. Hyattsville, MD: National Center for Health Statistics.

Vig, E., & Pearlman, R. (2004). Good and bad dying from the perspective of terminally ill men. *Archives of Internal Medicine, 164*(9), 977-981.

von Strauss, E., Agüero-Torres, H., Kåreholt, I., Winblad, B., & Fratiglioni, L. (2003, July). Women are more disabled in basic activities of daily living than men only in very advanced ages: A study on disability, morbidity, and mortality from the Kungsholmen Project. *Journal of Clinical Epidemiology, 56*(7), 669-77.

Weindruch, R. (1996). The retardation of aging by caloric restriction: Studies in rodents and primates. *Toxicologic Pathology, 24*(6), 742-745.

Weitzen, S., Teno, J. M., Fennell, M., & Mor, V. (2003, February). Factors associated with site of death: A national study of where people die. *Medical Care, 41*(2), 323-335.

Wenzlow, A. T., & Lipson, D. J. (2009). *Transitioning Medicaid enrollees from institutions to the community: Number of people eligible and number of transitions targeted under MFP. National evaluation of the Money Follows the Person (MFP) Demonstration Grant Program: Reports from the field #1.* Princeton, NJ: Mathematica Policy Research.

Whitaker, A. (2009). Family involvement in the institutional eldercare context. Towards a new understanding. *Journal of Aging Studies, 23*(3), 158-167.

White, K. M. (2002). Longevity advances in high-income countries, 1955-96. *Population and Development Review, 28*(1), 59-76.

Williams, G. C. (1957). Pleiotropy, natural selection, and the evolution of senescence. *Evolution, 11*(4), 398-411.

Wilmoth, J. R., & Lundstrom, H. (1996). Extreme longevity in five countries. *European Journal of Population, 12*, 63-93.

Wolf, R., Daichman, L., & Bennett, G. (2002). Abuse of the elderly. In E. G. Krug, L. L. Dahlberg, J. A. Mercy, A. B. Zwi, & R. Lozano (Eds.), *World Report on Violence and Health (pp.* 125-145). Geneva, Switzerland: World Health Organization.

SLEEP AND HEALTH

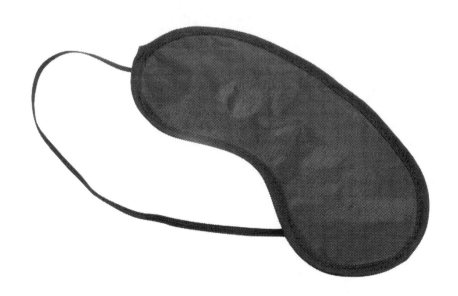

S leep is a necessary part of a healthy life and an essential aspect of health promotion and chronic disease prevention. Sufficient sleep is a vital sign of optimal well-being and not a luxury to be taken for granted. Unfortunately, a large number of individuals suffer from sleep disorders and related health issues. The National Institutes of Health (NIH) estimates that 50 to 70 million Americans are affected by chronic sleep complaints. Prior to the last decade, the loss of sleep was not considered a health risk. Current research has demonstrated that sleep disorders are associated with a host of health issues, such as mood and anxiety disorders, diabetes mellitus, increased blood pressure, and coronary heart disease (Ayas et al., 2003; Bjorvatn et al., 2007; Gottlieb et al., 2005; Hammond, 1964; Kripke, Garfinkel, Wingard, Klauber, & Marler, 2002; Leproult, Copinschi, Buxton, & Van Cauter, 1997; Spiegel, Leproult, & Van Cauter, 1999). Moreover, the effects of sleep disorders can cause impairments in daily activities, such as work, school, and leisure. Sleep disorder prevention recommendations entail following some simple sleep hygiene tips and seeking out a doctor or sleep specialist for accurate diagnosis and treatment. In addition, prioritizing sleep and incorporating the right amount of sleep each night into one's schedule is imperative for optimal health and functioning.

Sociocultural Influences

The discussion of sleep has evolved over thousands of years and sleep habits are continually adjusted to conform to societal norms and technological advances. Until recent decades, sleep was considered to be a prolonged state of not being awake. Now it is known that many vital tasks are carried out during sleep to help maintain good health and enable people to function at their best (National Institutes of Health, National Center on Sleep Disorder Research, 2008). Although society has changed, human brains and bodies have not. Sleep issues affect a large portion of the American population and consequences arise with disorders of this most basic human need (National Sleep Foundation, 2009). Unfortunately, the pace of life in Western society is fast and demanding, and sleep does not always fit into busy and hectic schedules.

Before artificial light was widely used, sleep was more closely tied to the schedule of the sun. People typically slept in two rounds called *first sleep* and *second sleep*. After the sun went down, people would go to sleep for approximately 4 hours and then get up to do household chores, visit with friends, and participate in other more leisure-like activities. They would then return to sleep at approximately 2 a.m. and sleep until sunrise. Historical documents show that *two sleeps* was widely known and practiced, and in some current cultures that do not have artificial light, it continues to be practiced (Ekirch, 2006). One study exposed a group of individuals to an artificial environment that mimicked the natural light/dark schedule and the participants began to revert to sleeping in two bouts just like in times before widely used artificial illumination (Wehr, 1992).

Currently, getting a good night's sleep is considered to consist of approximately 7 to 8 hours of uninterrupted sleep. Studies in Europe and the United States show that the amount of sleep individuals get now is 2 hours less than people 50 years ago (Kronholm et al., 2008; Van Cauter E., Leproult, R. & Plat, L., 2000). On average, adults in America are sleeping 6.8 hours a night on weekdays and 7.4 hours a night on weekends. Overall, adults in America report sleeping an average of 6.9 hours a night, when considering both weekday and weekend sleep. About one half of adults (49%) report having "a good night's sleep" every night or almost every night. In contrast, 26% report having "a good night's sleep" only a few nights a month or less and 24% report having "a good night's sleep" a few nights a week (National Sleep Foundation, 2005).

Sleep deprivation can be extremely dangerous. Individuals experiencing sleep deprivation that were tested using a driving simulator were found to perform as badly as or worse than participants who were intoxicated. Sleep deprivation has also been shown to increase the effect of alcohol on the body, so a fatigued person who drinks will become much more impaired than someone who is well rested (National Sleep Foundation, 2009). Driver fatigue is responsible for an estimated 100,000 motor vehicle accidents, 1,500 deaths each year, and costs Americans $12.5 billion per year in reduced productivity and property loss (National Highway Traffic Safety Administration, n.d.). Since drowsiness is the brain's last step before falling asleep, driving while drowsy can lead to disaster. Caffeine and other stimulants cannot overcome the effects of severe sleep deprivation (American Sleep Association, n.d.). Indications of sleep deprivation include, difficulty keeping the eyes focused, incessant yawning, and losing track of the past stretch of road that was driven. If an individual is experiencing these symptoms, they are most likely too drowsy to drive safely.

Biology and Physiology

Studies indicate that sleep has an ancient origin and appears to be homeostatically regulated like eating is (i.e., the body has a hunger mechanism that is triggered when one needs to eat). This is an indication that sleep is biologically controlled and a very important function for survival. Being awake, alert, and functional uses up fuel. The human body senses when that fuel has been depleted and triggers the urge to sleep, so the body can recover the energy needed to be awake again (Allada & Siegel, 2008). Sleep is also important because it facilitates the storage of new information into long-term memory (Born, Rasch, & Gais, 2006; Walker & Stickgold, 2004).

There are five distinct stages of sleep that can be measured: one stage of rapid eye movement (REM) sleep and four stages of non-rapid eye movement (NREM) sleep. Stage 1 of NREM sleep is the transition from being awake to being asleep and takes up about 5% of the time spent sleeping in healthy adults. Stage 2 of NREM composes about 50% of one's sleep. And stages 3 and 4 of NREM sleep (slow-wave sleep) are the deepest levels of sleep and compose about 10%-20% of time asleep. REM sleep, during which the majority of story-like dreams occur, is about 20%-25% of total sleep time. These stages do not happen in sequence throughout the night. Instead, NREM stages 3 and 4 usually occur in the first one third to one half of the night and will increase with sleep deprivation. REM tends to alternate with NREM sleep about every 80-100 minutes, and REM periods of sleep increase in frequency toward the morning, resulting in more memorable and vivid dreams. Also important to consider is that changes in sleep occur across a lifespan. Individuals need more slow-wave sleep in childhood and early adolescence because it is a time of physical growth and more sleep is required. As individuals get older, they need less sleep and the sleep cycle consists of more time in stage 1 of the transition from being awake to being asleep and less time in stages 3 and 4, which are the deepest of all the sleep stages.

In addition to the NREM and REM cycles, a circadian sleep-wake cycle controls bodily rhythms affecting sleep, such as melatonin levels and body temperature. This circadian cycle is triggered by outside factors such as light and social cues, like mealtimes and school or work schedules. A main component of the cycle is the *pineal gland*, which secretes the hormone melatonin. Melatonin plays a role in connecting the sleep-wake cycle to the light-dark cycle. With the retina triggering the process, melatonin is secreted the most during dark hours and the least in the daylight hours. The circadian clock gene can affect whether an individual is either a *morning type*, or *lark*, or an *evening type*, or *owl*. Owls are more susceptible to developing what is called *delayed sleep phase syndrome*. Delayed sleep phase syndrome results in sleep onset occurring in the early hours of the morning, making it difficult to wake up in the morning for school, work, or other important morning tasks. This is especially prominent in adolescence when there is an increased need for sleep and a tendency to go to bed later and a requirement to wake up earlier (Zaiwalla, 2004).

Sleep Disorder Classification

The *DSM-IV-TR* (American Psychiatric Association [APA], 2000) organizes sleep disorders into four major sections according to the origins of the disorder (i.e., whether biological in origin or due to other external factors). The first section is comprised of primary sleep disorders, which are explained by biological abnormalities in the sleep-wake or sleep timing mechanisms and are often complicated by behavioral factors, such as not having a reasonable sleep schedule. Primary sleep disorders are subdivided into *dyssomnias* and *parasomnias*. Dyssomnias are characterized by abnormalities in the amount, quality, or timing of sleep (e.g., insomnia). Parasomnias are characterized by abnormal behavior or physiological events occurring in association with sleep, specific sleep stages, or sleep-wake transitions (e.g., sleep walking). The second section of disorders is comprised of sleep disorders related to another mental disorder, such as insomnia associated with depression or anxiety. The third section is sleep disorders due to a general medical condition (e.g., a brain disorder that disrupts the physiological functions of normal sleep). The fourth section of sleep disorders is substance-induced sleep disorders (e.g., consuming too much caffeine or taking illicit drugs).

Dyssomnias
Insomnia. Insomnia is characterized by one or more of the following: difficulty initiating sleep, difficulty maintaining sleep, waking up too early, and/or sleep that is chronically non-restorative or of poor quality (APA, 2000). Individuals with insomnia have been shown to experience an increased risk for psychiatric disorders, such as major depressive disorder, anxiety, and substance abuse. It is also associated with decreased quality of life, increased healthcare use, and decreased productivity (Roth, 2009; Roth, Franklin, & Bramley, 2007). Insomnia is nearly twice as common in women than in men,

and women are more likely than men to report insomnia to their healthcare professional (APA, 2000).

Hypersomnia. Hypersomnia is characterized by excessive sleepiness for at least a month that is sufficient enough to impair normal everyday functioning (APA, 2000).

Sleep apnea syndromes and snoring. Sleep apnea syndromes and snoring effect nearly 40% of the U.S. population and half of the cases are clinically significant and warrant treatment (Dement, 1999). Sleep apnea is defined as the absence of airflow for 10 or more seconds during sleep (Lee-Chiong, 2008, p. 37). When airflow is reduced but not totally absent, it is called *hypopnea*. During sleep apnea, airflow is restricted or reduced and the muscles of the diaphragm struggle to breath against the blocked throat. Carbon dioxide builds up in the bloodstream and oxygen is reduced. The individual struggles to breathe and, with a series of gasps and snores, breathing starts over again. Individuals suffering from sleep apnea are not aware that they have stopped breathing and remain asleep. After beginning to breathe again, snoring begins, as does the cycle, repeating hundreds of times a night (Dement, 1999). Sleep apnea tends to start appearing in both men and women in their 30s, 40s, or 50s. The overall prevalence in men is 1 in 4, and the prevalence of sleep apnea in women is lower until after menopause when they nearly equal the rates of men (Dement, 1999). Obstructive sleep apnea (OSA), central sleep apnea (CSA), and mixed central and obstructive apnea are the major classifications of sleep apnea syndromes. OSA is the most common and affects at least 5% of the population and some studies estimate that even 20% of the adult population suffers from OSA (Lee-Chiong, 2008).

Narcolepsy. Narcolepsy is a sleep disorder that causes individuals to fall asleep during inappropriate times. It is more complicated and much less prominent than other sleep disorders with prevalence estimates approximately 0.02% to 0.16% in the U.S. adult population, or about 25 in every 100,000 people. Narcolepsy is defined as having an irresistible urge to sleep daily for at least three months that must be accompanied by brief moments of having no muscle control and/or experiencing REM sleep during the first stages of falling asleep (REM sleep is not supposed to occur until later in the sleep cycle).

Circadian rhythm sleep disorder. Circadian rhythm sleep disorder is characterized by individuals that have difficulty matching their own internal biological sleep rhythms to the external demands of their schedule. This mismatch can result in insomnia at times and hypersomnia at other times. There are three subtypes identified within the disorder. *Delayed sleep phase type* occurs when a person naturally and habitually falls asleep late at night and has extreme difficulty waking up in the morning for daily activities, often needing multiple alarm clocks. These individuals experience normal sleep once they are asleep, but the problem is that their bodies are not in sync with their social and/or work schedules. For example, a person who is biologically predisposed to being a "night person" but is forced to wake up early in the morning for work. *Jet lag type* is one of the more familiar disorders and is rarely a chronic concern unless one is traveling through different time zones on a frequent basis. *Shift work type* occurs when an individual is forced to work a schedule that is in conflict with their biological sleep pattern (APA, 2000).

Parasomnias

Nightmare disorder. Nightmare disorder is characterized by repeated occurrences of frightening dreams that wake up an individual. The individual becomes fully alert upon awakening, and the dreams or sleep interruptions disrupt the individual's daily life and cause significant stress. Nightmares can result in insomnia, avoiding sleep due to being fearful of nightmares, excessive sleepiness during the day, and anxiety. Nightmares can be precipitated by illness, traumatic experiences, drinking alcohol, and taking certain medications. Having occasional nightmares is common and most people who experience them do not have any underlying mental disorder. It is estimated that 10%-50% of children report having nightmares and experience a peak from ages 6-10 years old (Lee-Chiong, 2008).

Sleep terror disorder. Sleep terror disorder is characterized by experiencing abrupt awakenings from sleep usually beginning with a panicky scream or cry lasting for 1-10 minutes, acting out physically to the intense fear, and difficulty waking up or being comforted. Dream recall is minimal.

Sleep walking disorder. Sleep walking disorder is characterized by repeated episodes of complex movements during sleep (e.g., getting out of bed and walking around) that occur during the first third of the night, reduced awareness of actions, a blank stare, an inability to respond to arousal if woken up, very limited recall of the episode, and difficulty with re-orientation after the episode. These episodes cause significant problems in a person's life.

Treatment

Behavioral treatments can be effective for people who are highly motivated and practice the techniques that are given to them. Behavioral treatments require the assistance of a practitioner, and it is important for the patient to realize that these techniques take time to work (Buysse, 2008). One of the major problems with behavioral therapies is not that they do not work but that there is often a lack of clinician awareness and adequate training in the skills needed to treat patients (Benca, 2005). Some behavioral changes, such as keeping a regular sleep schedule, exercise, stress reduction, avoiding smoking and alcohol, and restricting the use of certain medications, can assist in reducing sleep problems.

Most sleep disorders are treated with a combination of behavioral therapy and medication. Benzodiazepines are a class of medication very commonly prescribed for many sleep disorders; however, long-term use is somewhat controversial. The U.S. Food and Drug Administration (FDA) labeling states, "Hypnotics should generally be limited to seven to ten days of use, and reevaluation of the patient is recommended if they are to be taken for more than two to three weeks. [The drug] should not be prescribed in quantities exceeding a one-month supply" (as cited in *Physicians' Desk Reference (PDR)*, 2003). There is evidence that the majority of medications used for sleep can produce tolerance or dependence in patients ("Chat Transcript," n.d.). For a person using medication every night or nearly every night, the medication may eventually lose effectiveness or the person may become reliant on the medication. The decision to use benzodiazepines must be arrived at with doctor approval and after all other methods have been attempted (Appleton, 2004). Sleep specialist Dr. Lauren Broch (2008) points out that research shows the "behavioral changes that we make are much more effective and long-lasting than taking a medication on a regular basis." There are also non-benzodiazepine medications that may be prescribed for disorders that work very similarly to benzodiazepines but may have fewer side effects. Sedating anti-depressants, the most coming being Trazadone, are also often used to treat certain sleep disorders (Lavie, Pillar, & Malhotra, 2002).

The treatment of sleep apnea disorders necessitates the use of positive airway pressure therapy and consists of a particular machine that controls breathing for the patient. There are 4 general types of positive airway pressure devices: (1) continuous positive airway pressure (CPAP), (2) bilevel positive airway pressure (BiPAP), (3) autotitrating positive airway pressure (APAP), and (4) adaptive servo ventilation (Lee-Chiong, 2008).

Complementary and Alternative Treatments

The use of herbal medicine in the US has been growing since the 1994 Dietary and Supplement Health and Education Act, which put herbs into their own category of regulation called *dietary supplements*. Dietary supplements can make claims that they are *helpful* for medical issues but cannot claim that they *prevent* or *treat* disease (Eisenberg et al., 1998). Herbal supplements come in a wide variety of forms to choose from, such as teas, tinctures (liquid extracts of herbs), and capsules. It is wise to be informed concerning the efficacy of some of the herbal concoctions promoted to help sleep or sleepiness. The following are commonly used and marketed herbal supplements for sleep and sleepiness:

Caffeine and caffeine-containing herbs. Caffeine is a mild stimulant and a natural chemical found in the leaves, seeds, or fruits of more that 60 plant species worldwide (Gyllenhall, Merritt, Peterson, Block, & Gochenour, 2000). Plants containing caffeine are often used in beverages, such as coffee and tea and other varieties like kola, guarana, and mate. Some energy drinks incorporate different types of caffeine-containing herbs and have more caffeine than most sodas (Grand & Bell, 1997). Caffeine use has been shown to typically contribute to lack of sleep. However, for some people, it is possible for them to consume caffeine and not have sleeping difficulties. This may be due to people adjusting their caffeine intake to work with their sleep schedule or certain individuals possibly reacting to caffeine in different ways and not experiencing sleep problems (Pantelios, Lack, & James, 1989). Unfortunately, a paucity of research on the caffeine use of people with sleep disorders exists; however, anecdotally, it has been noted that it is by no means unusual for those suffering from sleep problems to use caffeine to battle daytime sleepiness (Gyllenhall et al., 2000).

Ephedra-containing herbs. Ephedra is a plant derivative and was one of the first drugs used to treat narcolepsy (Mitler, Aldrich, Koob, & Zarcone, 1994). Traditionally used to treat asthma and congestion, it is now used for energy, weight loss, and some bodybuilding products (Gyllenhall et al., 2000). Adverse effects, such as tachycardia, anxiety, tremor, insomnia, seizure, and other similar issues, have been found with using ephedra alkaloids. The FDA (2008) identifies ephedrine alkaloids as "an unreasonable risk of illness or injury under the conditions of use recommended or suggested in labeling, or if no conditions of use are suggested or recommended in labeling, under ordinary conditions of use." Therefore, it is imperative to take precautions while using ephedra and consult a physician if planning on usage.

Yohimbe bark. Yohimbe bark is a traditional aphrodisiac used in African countries but has been used to treat the intense urge to nap associated with narcolepsy (Poceta, Hajdukovic, & Mitler, 1994).

Ginseng. There are various types of ginseng. Panax ginseng was traditionally used in Chinese medicine to fight fatigue and stress.

Limited and conflicting studies have been conducted on the anti-fatigue properties of Panax ginseng, and adverse effects have been observed in some studies (Gyllenhall et al., 2000).

Valerian. In Europe, valerian has been widely used since the 17th century for its sedative properties. Valerian has benzodiazepine-like effects on the brain. To determine valerian's effectiveness as a sleep aid, studies on humans have been performed, and positive results have been recorded (Gyllenhall et al., 2000).

German chamomile. The sedative effects of chamomile are mild and there is a lack of extensive research on chamomile's efficacy as a sleep aid. However, one small study did show that chamomile was effective in inducing sleep (Gould, Reddy, & Comprecht, 1973).

Kava-kava. Kava-kava has recently begun to be used to treat anxiety and sleep disorders in the United States and Europe (Schulz, Hansel, & Tyler, 1998). Studies have demonstrated that kava-kava does help people sleep and could possibly be helpful for people that suffer from anxiety-related sleep disturbances (Emser & Bartylla, 1991; Klimke, Klieser, Lehmann, & Strauss, 1989).

Lavender. Lavender is usually used in oil form and is inhaled to induce sleepiness. Studies have indicated that it is effective in inducing sleepiness and even improved sleep quality (Buchbauer, Jirovetz, Jäger, Dietrich, & Plank, 1991; Hardy, Kirk-Smith, & Stretch, 1995).

Prevention

Having a regular sleep schedule and keeping the environment one sleeps in quiet and at a comfortable temperature are two practices that can aid disordered sleep behavior. Also, new methods for assessing and treating sleeplessness are being improved, indicating progress toward relief for millions suffering from sleep problems (CDC, 2011). Prevention of sleep disorders starts with *sleep hygiene*, the habits that contribute to healthy sleep patterns. Lifestyle changes to accommodate better sleep hygiene can keep a person from developing a sleep disorder. In addition, a general healthy lifestyle, such as eating the right foods, exercising, and reducing stress, is very important for the prevention of sleep problems.

We interviewed Paul, a 70-year-old, for a personal perspective on living with a sleep disorder. Paul's sleep disorder escalated to the point where he was falling asleep while driving his truck during the day. He would be forced to stop and take naps. Being tired became a problem for Paul and his wife. Paul would wake his wife with the sound of his snoring and when his snoring would stop because he would also stop breathing then. Paul's wife would have to nudge him repeatedly to restart his breathing.

Using a CPAP (continuous positive airway pressure) machine allowed the couple to sleep again. They can now sleep through most nights and have better days. Paul believes there is no way not to succeed with a CPAP unless it doesn't fit properly, in which case it can be adjusted or another one can be tried. He and his wife strongly recommend the CPAP and wish to convince others to try it.

For a personal account of dealing with a sleep disorder, we interviewed Sheila, a 27-year-old woman. Sheila suffers from nightmares four to five times per week. Some challenges she faces from this disorder are waking up feeling stressed, anxious, and tired and having a lack of energy for the rest of the day. Shelia has used meditation and chamomile tea to help her relax before going to sleep and aid in avoiding nightmares. She believes they have been successful because she has noticed a difference in her sleep and nightmare patterns when they are used. The relaxation methods do reduce the number of nights Sheila has nightmares per week, but they do not always work for her. Sheila suggests that others with a sleep disorder try to find methods for coping that work for them. She also recommends they seek professional help.

Conclusion

When sleep becomes disordered, it can be very disruptive to one's life and contribute to a host of medical and mental health issues. At times it may seem there are not enough hours in the day to accomplish everything that needs to be accomplished and still have time to rest. Sleep disorders are becoming more common and many individuals suffer from issues regarding this most basic human need. As individuals continue to get less and less sleep and the demands of bustling and busy lives cause increased stress and time commitments, disorders may become more the norm than the exception. Fortunately, many resources are available for individuals suffering from sleep problems. However, the best remedy for the majority of sleep complaints is actually getting the amount of sleep needed.

Recommendations

The following are guidelines to good sleep hygiene from the U.S. Department of Health and Human Services, National Institutes of Health, National Heart, Lung, and Blood Institute (2006):

A good sleep environment:
- Dark. Avoid lights, including night-lights. Keep the windows covered with blinds or curtains.
- Cool. Keep the temperature of the sleep environment cool enough to necessitate blankets for warmth.
- Quiet. Falling asleep and staying asleep is much easier if the environment is quiet. Use earplugs or a "white noise machine" if it is difficult to control the noise level in the sleep environment.
- Comfortable. A comfortable mattress that provides back support and will not contribute to stiffness and soreness in the morning.

A good night's sleep:
- An uninterrupted sleep
- A refreshing sleep
- A deep sleep
- A length of time that works for an individual personally (the average adult needs 7.5 to 8 hours per night).

Barriers to a good night's sleep:

- Consuming alcohol before bed. Alcohol may make it easier to fall asleep but it is at the cost of quality. Alcohol fragments sleep, so an individual will not feel well rested even after a full night of sleep.
- Certain medications. Some medications have side effects associated with insomnia. This is also the case for certain herbal remedies. Make sure to read the accompanying informational material and to consult a doctor or pharmacist before using these products.

How to get a good night's sleep:

- Have a bedtime ritual. This sends a cue to the body that it is time to settle down and fall asleep. A ritual does not have to be a long process and can be as simple as brushing your teeth and reading for 15 minutes.
- Keep a regular sleeping pattern. This allows the body's biological clock to set an internal alarm for bedtime and ensures that one will be alert during the appropriate times of the day. One way to set the biological clock is to sit in the direct sun for 15 minutes right after waking up in the morning, which prompts the body to tune in to the time of day.
- Have a light snack before bed. This allows for sound sleep through the night without waking up from hunger pangs. Be careful with portions: eating a heavy meal before going to bed will make it difficult to fall asleep.
- Unwind earlier in the evening. Take the time early in the evening to relax the body and mind. Falling asleep can be almost impossible if one's mind is racing, working through problems, weighing decisions and reviewing the past day or upcoming events and responsibilities. A calm, clear mind is necessary for a relaxed body.
- Take a warm bath before going to bed. Warm baths raise the body's temperature. After the bath the body cools off and this cooling process induces sleepiness.

Barriers to the transition to sleep:

- Staying up too late. By staying up too late one is liable to get a "second wind," which will make it difficult to fall asleep even if it is late.
- Eating a large or heavy meal before bed. Heartburn, indigestion, and the need to urinate are counterproductive and end up disturbing sleep.
- Doing things other than sleeping in bed (watching TV, working, etc.). If an individual engages in activities other than sleep (or sex) in bed, the brain will cease to recognize cues indicating that bed is the place for sleep.
- Having caffeine before bed. Caffeine is a stimulant that can keep the body awake and alert.
- Cigarette smoking. The nicotine found in cigarettes is a stimulant and will interfere with the body's ability to fall asleep.
- Exercising directly before bedtime. Exercise is healthy and can be very helpful if it is done several hours before going to sleep. Exercising before bedtime will inhibit sleep because of the natural high produced from exercise.
- Trying to force the body to fall asleep. If an individual cannot fall asleep after 30 minutes, it is wise to get up and do something that is not stimulating. Forcing oneself to lie in bed will only be frustrating and take one even farther from the goal of sleep.
- Daytime naps. Avoid daytime naps because they stagger the body's biological rhythm. By taking naps, one may not be tired at bedtime and this will encourage a later bedtime. If an individual doesn't go to bed at a reasonable hour, they might feel tired the next day and opt for another daytime nap, which establishes a vicious cycle. If napping is necessary, sleep for less than 1 hour before 3 p.m.

Selected Resources

American Academy of Sleep Medicine (AASM)
One Westbrook Corporate Center, Suite 920
Westchester, IL 60154
708-492-0930; Fax: 708-492-0943
www.aasmnet.org

American Insomnia Association
One Westbrook Corporate Center, Suite 920
Westchester, IL 60154
708-492-0930
rmoney@aasmnet.org
www.americaninsomniaassociation.org

American Sleep Apnea Association
1424 K Street, NW, Suite 302
Washington, DC 20005
202-293-3650; Fax: 202-293-3656
www.sleepapnea.org

Narcolepsy Network, Inc.
P.O. Box 294
Pleasantville, NY 10570
401-667-2523; Fax: 401-633-6567
narnet@narcolepsynetwork.org
www.narcolepsynetwork.org

National Center on Sleep Disorders Research
National Heart, Lung, and Blood Institute, NIH
6701 Rockledge Drive
Bethesda, MD 20892-7993
301-435-0199; Fax: 301-480-3451
ncsdr@nih.gov
www.nhlbi.nih.gov/sleep

National Sleep Foundation
1522 K Street, NW, Suite 500
Washington, DC 20005
202-347-3471; Fax: 202-347-3472
nsf@sleepfoundation.org
www.sleepfoundation.org

NHLBI Health Information Center
P.O. Box 30105
Bethesda, MD 20824-0105
301-592-8573; TTY: 240-629-3255; Fax: 301-592-8563
nhlbiinfo@nhlbi.nih.gov
www.nhlbi.nih.gov

References

Allada, R., & Siegel, M. (2008, August 5). Unearthing the phylogenetic roots of sleep. *Current Biology, 18*, 670-679.

American Psychiatric Association. (2000). *Diagnostic and statistical manual of mental disorders* (Revised 4th ed.). Washington, DC: Author.

American Sleep Association (n.d.). Patients/General Public [Internet]. Retrieved from http://sleepassociation.org/index.php?p=patients.

Appleton, W. S. (2004). *The new anti-depressants and anti-anxieties: What you need to know about Zoloft, Paxil, Wellbutrin, Effexor, Clonazepam, Ambien, and more.* New York, NY: Plume Books.

Ayas, N. T., White, D. P., Manson, J. E., Stampfer, M. J., Speizer, F. E., Malhotra, A., & Hu, F. B. (2003). A prospective study of sleep duration and coronary heart disease in women. *Archives of Internal Medicine, 163*, 205-209.

Benca, R. M. (2005). Diagnosis and treatment of chronic insomnia: A review. *Psychiatric Services, 56*, 332-343.

Bjorvatn, B., Sagen, I. M., Øyane, N., Waage, S., Fetveit, A., Pallesen, S., & Ursin, R. (2007). The association between sleep duration, body mass index and metabolic measures in the Hordaland Health Study. *Journal of Sleep Research, 16*(1), 66-76.

Born, J., Rasch, B., & Gais, S. (2006). Sleep to remember. *The Neuroscientist, 12*, 410-424.

Broch, L. (2008, August 24). Insomnia prevention [Blog post]. Retrieved from http://stanford.wellsphere.com/insomnia-sleep-disorders-article/insomnia-prevention/79646

Buchbauer, G., Jirovetz, L., Jäger, W., Dietrich, H., & Plank, C. (1991). Aromatherapy: Evidence for sedative effects of the essential oil of lavender after inhalation. *Zeithschrift fur Naturforschung, 46*(11-12), 1067-1072.

Buysse, D. (2008, August 24). Gaining control over sleep problems [Blog post]. Retrieved from http://stanford.wellsphere.com/insomnia-sleep-disorders-article/gaining-control-over-sleep-problems/79928

Centers for Disease Control and Prevention. (2011). Sleep and sleep disorders. Retrieved March 18, 2011, from http://www.cdc.gov/sleep/index.htm

Chat transcript: Dr. Clete Kushida on sleep disorders. (n.d.). Retrieved September 20, 2009, from http://www.cnn.com/HEALTH/9910/05/chat.kushida.sleep/index.html

Dement, W. (1999). *The promise of sleep.* New York, NY: Delacorte Press.

Eisenberg, D. M., Davis, R. B., Ettner, S. L., Appel, S., Wilkey, S., Van Rompay, M., & Kessler, R. C. (1998). Trends in alternative medicine use in the United States, 1990-1997: Results of a follow-up national survey. *Journal of the American Medical Association, 280*(18), 1569-1575.

Ekirch, A. R. (2006). *At day's close: Night in times past.* New York, NY: Norton.

Emser, W., & Bartylla, K. (1991). Improvement in sleep quality. Effect of kava extract WS 1490 on the sleep pattern in healthy subjects [in German, English abstract]. *Neurology and Psychiatry, 5,* 636-642.

Gottlieb, D. J., Punjabi, N. M., Newman, A. B., Resnick, H. E., Redline, S., Baldwin, C. M., & Nieto, F. J. (2005). Association of sleep time with diabetes mellitus and impaired glucose tolerance. *Archives of Internal Medicine, 165,* 863-867.

Gould, L., Reddy, C. V. R., & Comprecht, R. F. (1973). Cardiac effect of chamomile tea. *Journal of Clinical Pharmacology, 13,* 475-479.

Grand, A. N., & Bell, L. N. (1997). Caffeine content of fountain and private-label store brand carbonated beverages. *Journal of American Dietetic Association, 97,* 179-182.

Gyllenhall, C., Merritt, S. L., Peterson, S. D., Block, K. I., & Gochenour, T. (2000). Efficacy and safety of herbal stimulants and sedatives in sleep disorders. *Sleep Medicine Reviews, 4*(3), 229-251.

Hammond, E. C. (1964). Some preliminary findings on physical complaints from a prospective study of 1,064,004 men and women. *American Journal of Public Health and the Nations Health, 54,* 11-23.

Hardy, M., Kirk-Smith, M., & Stretch, D. (1995) Replacement of drug treatment for insomnia by ambient odour. *Lancet, 346,* 701.

Klimke, A., Klieser, E., Lehmann, E., & Strauss, W. H. (1989). The clinical efficacy of kavain in the treatment of anxiety syndromes in comparison with other anxiolytics. *Pharmacopsychiatry, 22,* 201-202.

Kripke, D. F., Garfinkel, L., Wingard, D. L., Klauber, M. R., &

Marler, M. R. (2002). Mortality associated with sleep duration and insomnia. *Archives of General Psychiatry, 59*, 131-136.

Kronholm, E. (2008). Trends in self-reported sleep duration and insomnia-related symptoms in Finland from 1972 to 2005: a comparative review and re-analysis of Finnish population samples. *Journal of Sleep Research, 17*(1), 54–62.

Lavie, P., Pillar, A., & Malhotra, A. (Eds.). (2002). *Sleep disorders: Diagnosis, management, and treatment. A handbook for clinicians.* London, England: Dunitz.

Lee-Chiong, T. (2008). *Sleep medicine: Essentials and review.* New York, NY: Oxford University Press.

Leproult, R., Copinschi, G., Buxton, O., & Van Cauter, E. (1997). Sleep loss results in an elevation of cortisol levels the next evening. *Sleep, 20*, 865-870.

Mitler, M., Aldrich, M. S., Koob, G. F., & Zarcone, V. P. (1994). Narcolepsy and its treatment with stimulants. ASDA standards of practice. *Sleep, 17*(4), 352-371.

National Highway Traffic Safety Administration. (n.d.) *Drowsy driving and automobile crashes: NCSDR/NHTSA expert panel on driver fatigue and sleepiness.* Retrieved from http://www.nhtsa.dot.gov/PEOPLE/INJURY/drowsy_driving1/drowsy.html

National Institutes of Health (2008). National Center on Sleep Disorder Research. Retrieved September 20, 2009, from http://www.nhlbi.nih.gov/about/ncsdr/index.htm

National Sleep Foundation. (2005). 2005 Sleep in America Poll. Retrieved September 20, 2009, from http://www.sleepfoundation.org/article/sleep-america-polls/2005-adult-sleep-habits-and-styles

National Sleep Foundation. (2009). 2009 Sleep in America Poll. Retrieved September 20, 2009, from http://www.sleepfoundation. org/article/sleep-america-polls/2009-health-and safety

Pantelios, G., Lack, L., & James, J. (1989). Caffeine consumption and sleep. *Sleep Research, 18,* 65-72.

Physicians' desk reference (57th ed.). (2003). Montvale, NJ: Thomson.

Poceta, J. S., Hajdukovic, R., & Mitler, M. M. (1994). Improvement in cataplexy with yohimbe and paroxetine: Case report. *Sleep Research, 23,* 304.

Roth, T. (2009, February). Comorbid insomnia: Current directions and future challenges. *American Journal of Managed Care, 15*(1), S6-S13.

Roth, T., Franklin, M., & Bramley, T. J. (2007). The state of insomnia and emerging trends. *The American Journal of Managed Care, 13*(5), S117-S120.

Schulz, V., Hansel, R., & Tyler, V. E. (1998). *Rational phytotherapy: A physicians' guide to herbal medicine* (3rd ed.). Berlin, Germany: Springer-Verlag.

Spiegel, K., Leproult, R., & Van Cauter, E. (1999). Impact of sleep debt on metabolic and endocrine function. *Lancet, 354,* 1435-1439.

U.S. Department of Health and Human Services, National Institutes of Health, National Heart, Lung, and Blood Institute. (2006). *In brief: Your guide to healthy sleep* (NIH Publication No. 06-5800). Retrieved from http://www.nhlbi.nih.gov/health/ public/sleep /healthysleepfs.pdf

U. S. Food and Drug Administration. (2008). *Guidance for industry: Final rule declaring dietary supplements containing ephedrine alkaloids adulterated because they present an unreasonable risk; Small entity compliance guide.* Retrieved October 20, 2009, from http://www.fda.gov/Food/GuidanceComplianceRegulatoryInformation/GuidanceDocuments/DietarySupplements/ucm072997.htm

Van Cauter, E., Leproult, R., & Plat, L. (2000). Age-related changes in slow wave sleep and REM sleep and relationship with growth hormone and cortisol levels in healthy men. *Journal of the American Medical Association, 284*(7), 861-868.

Walker, M. P., & Stickgold, R. (2004). Sleep-dependent learning review and memory consolidation. *Neuron, 44*, 121-133.

Wehr, T. A. (1992). In short photoperiods, human sleep is biphasic. *Journal of Sleep Research, 1*, 103-107.

Zaiwalla, Z. (2004, June 13). Dealing with abnormal sleep patterns. *Pulse.* Retrieved from http://www.pulsetoday.co.uk/main-content/-/article_display_list/10889103/dealing-with-abnormal-sleep-patterns

MENTAL HEALTH

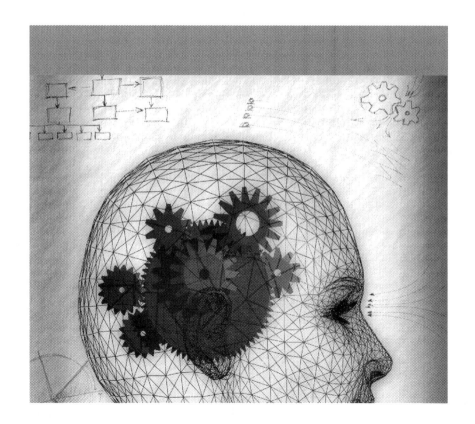

The World Health Organization (WHO) *defines* mental health as "a state of complete physical, mental and social well-being, and not merely the absence of disease" and *describes* mental health as "a state of well-being in which the individual realizes his or her own abilities, can cope with the normal amount of stresses of life, can work productively and fruitfully, and is able to make a contribution to his or her community" (Herrman, Saxena, & Moodie, 2005, p. XVII). Mental illness encompasses a range of medical conditions that "disrupt a person's thinking, feeling, mood, ability to relate to others and daily functioning" (National Alliance on Mental Illness [NAMI], n.d.). Serious mental illnesses include major depressive disorder, schizophrenia, bipolar disorder, obsessive-compulsive disorder (OCD), panic disorder, post-traumatic stress disorder, and personality disorders.

Mental disorders are common in the United States. Approximately one quarter of individuals are diagnosable for one or more disorders in a lifetime. Mental disorders are the leading cause of disability in the US and Canada for persons ages 15 to 44 (World Health Organization [WHO], 2004). Many people suffer from more than one mental disorder at a given time. Nearly half (45%) of those with any mental disorder meet criteria for two or more disorders (National Institute of Mental Health [NIMH], 2010b). Although mental disorders are widespread, the main burden of illness is concentrated among a much smaller proportion of the population (about 1 in 17 adults) who suffer from chronic and severe mental illness (NIMH, 2010a). Many determinants related to social, psychological, genetic, and biological factors contribute to the level of mental health of a person at any point in time. The genetic and biological contributors to mental illness are less understood than the other factors; however, continual research is conducted in this area and some genetic and biological features have been successfully identified as contributors to mental disorders.

Biology and Physiology

Neurology

Not all brain diseases are classified as mental illnesses. Disorders such as Parkinson's disease and multiple sclerosis are brain disorders, and they are considered neurological diseases as opposed to mental illnesses. However, as scientists continue to investigate the brains of mentally ill individuals, they are finding that mental disorders are linked with biology and are associated with the structure, chemistry, and function of the brain just like neurological disorders. This knowledge has contributed to scientists minimizing the distinction between mental illnesses and other brain disorders (NIMH, n.d.).

Many scientists studying mental illnesses believe they result from problematic communication between neurons in the brain. Individuals that experience depression have lower serotonin (a chemical produced in the brain that influences mood) levels than individuals not experiencing depression. These findings led to the development of selective serotonin reuptake inhibitors (SSRIs), which reduce the amount of serotonin that is consumed by the presynaptic neuron. This leads to an increase in the amount of serotonin available in the synaptic space for binding to the receptor on the postsynaptic neuron. Other neurotransmitters have been identified in addition to serotonin that may influence depression, adding to the complexity of the disorder. Disruptions in the neurotransmitters dopamine, glutamate, and norepinephrine have also been identified in individuals who have schizophrenia (NIMH, n.d.).

Substantial progress has been made in identifying and testing efficacious psychotherapeutic, somatic, and pharmacological interventions for many mental disorders. Nonetheless, the most current and effective interventions still fail to work for many individuals (Lennox, 2009). Virtually all approved drugs for mental illnesses have been variations on the compounds available four decades ago. The National Institute of Mental Health (NIMH) practical trials on pharmaceuticals for mental illness, such as the Clinical Antipsychotic Trials of Intervention Effectiveness (CATIE) and the Sequenced Treatment Alternatives to Relieve Depression (STAR*D) Study, document the limited effectiveness of the current medications and reveal the need for a new generation of medications for mental disorders. Key pharmaceutical companies have announced their intentions to move out of the business of psychiatric drug development, which raises the question of who will develop this next generation of treatments (NIMH, 2010b).

There is scarce literature to guide clinicians and patients in creating treatment strategies based on genetics, physiology, or behavioral characteristics so that individuals can receive personalized care (NIMH, 2010b). Given that half of all mentally ill adults report the onset of symptoms by the age of 14 and three quarters by their mid-20s (Kessler et al., 2005), it is increasingly apparent that locating the origins of mental disorders by identifying the mechanisms of brain structure and chemistry is an imperative next step in diagnosis and treatment, especially since symptoms may not indicate the onset of a disease and can appear long after the causal processes that lead to mental illness (NIMH, 2010b).

Current brain imaging technology allows for the investigation of mental illnesses and is being used increasingly to assist in research studies to learn about mental disorders; however, this technology does not have the capacity to assist in diagnosing an individual with a particular disorder. In some cases, a brain scan may be used to detect other medical illnesses, such as a tumor, that can cause symptoms similar to a mental disorder. Studies are also being conducted to compare the differences between the brains of people with and without mental illnesses to better understand these disorders. Some types of brain scans pose health risks due to the radiation involved and should not be done unless deemed necessary by a health official (U.S. Department of Health and Human Services, National Institutes of Health, NIMH, n.d.).

The two main types of neuroimaging, or brain scans, are (1) *structural imaging*, which creates a "snapshot" of the brain's structure, including bone, tissue, blood vessels, tumors, infection, damage, or bleeding such as from a stroke and (2) *functional imaging*, which reveals the brain's ever-changing activity and chemistry by measuring the rate of blood flow, chemical activity, and electrical impulses in the brain during specific tasks. Changes on structural imaging tests are seen in all the major psychiatric illnesses (schizophrenia, bipolar disorder, depression, and obsessive-compulsive disorder). Functional brain imaging is currently believed to have the true potential of helping in the near future with the diagnosis and treatment decisions for patients with mental illness (Lennox, 2009).

Genetics

In 2003, the Human Genome Project contributed to a growing optimism that psychiatric disorders could be identified through uncovering gene patterns. In subsequent years, some progress has been made toward understanding the relationship between heritability and mental illness (Barber, 2008). Illnesses such as bipolar disorder, depression, and schizophrenia are more likely to have a genetic component. Studies show that identical twins, when compared to fraternal twins, are more likely to share the aforementioned disorders. Also, studies indicate that individuals that have a parent or sibling with bipolar disorder, depression, or schizophrenia are more likely to suffer from the same mental disorder. No single gene has been found to trigger the onset of mental illness, and it is highly unlikely that one will ever be identified. Currently, mental disorders are believed to be a complex interaction of multiple genetic, environmental, and social factors (Barber, 2008; NIMH, n.d.).

Main Types of Mental Disorders

Depression

Depression has several forms, but the most common types are major depressive disorder, minor depression, and dysthymia. Major depressive disorder is characterized by a combination of symptoms such as an inability to work, sleep, study, eat, and enjoy pleasurable activities. These symptoms can be very disabling, preventing the person from functioning in everyday life. Dysthymic disorder is similar to major depressive disorder, but the symptoms are long term (2 years or longer) and tend to be less severe than those of major depression. Minor depression is also similar to major depression; however, it is less severe and for a shorter term. Other types of depression that can occur are psychotic depression and seasonal affective disorder (NIMH, 2010b).

Bipolar Disorder

Bipolar disorder is a brain disorder that causes shifts in mood, energy, and activity levels and affects the ability to function in everyday life (Kleinman et al., 2003). Individuals who suffer from bipolar disorder experience unusually intense emotional states that occur in distinct periods called *mood episodes*. Mood episodes are characterized by a manic episode (an overly joyful or excited state) and a depressive episode (an extremely sad or hopeless state). Sometimes a mood episode can consist of both, which is called a mixed state. People with bipolar disorder experience extreme changes in energy, activity, sleep, and behavior and can also be characterized by explosive anger and irritability. It is also possible for an individual to experience long-lasting periods of unstable moods as opposed to discreet episodes of mania or depression (NIMH, 2010b).

Anxiety Disorders

Anxiety disorders comprise a wide range of disorders, such as generalized anxiety disorder, obsessive-compulsive disorder, phobias, and post-traumatic stress disorder (NIMH, 2010b; WHO, 2004). Anxiety disorders are unlike the relatively mild and brief anxiety caused by a stressful event, last at least six months, and can get worse if not treated. Also, these disorders commonly occur with other mental or physical illnesses, such as substance or alcohol abuse, which can mask anxiety symptoms and even make them worse (NIMH, 2010b).

Eating Disorders

Eating disorders mainly occur in adolescent and adult females, especially ballet students, athletes, fashion models, and culinary students. The two main types of eating disorders are anorexia nervosa and bulimia nervosa. Anorexia nervosa is characterized by emaciation, a relentless pursuit of thinness, an unwillingness to maintain a healthy weight, a distortion of body image, an intense fear of gaining weight, a lack of menstruation in females, and disturbed eating behavior. Bulimia nervosa is characterized by binge-eating (frequent episodes of eating unusually large amounts of food) and feeling a lack of control over the eating, which is then followed by a compensatory behavior such as purging, fasting, and/or excessive exercise. Unlike with anorexia, individuals with bulimia are often within their normal weight range; however, like anorexics, bulimics fear gaining weight, pursue weight loss efforts, and are intensely unhappy with their body (NIMH, 2010b).

Psychotic Disorders

Psychotic disorders are severe mental disorders that cause abnormal thinking and perceptions. They also cause an individual to become detached from reality. Psychotic disorders include schizophrenia, schizoaffective disorder, delusional disorder, and other disorders characterized by similar symptomatology. The two main symptoms of psychotic disorders are (1) delusions—false beliefs, such as believing that characters in a television show are plotting against oneself and (2) hallucinations—false perceptions, such as hearing, seeing, or feeling something that is not actually there (NIMH, 2011). The onset of a psychotic disorder can be a potential disaster and have far-reaching consequences in many aspects of one's life (WHO, 2004).

Personality Disorders

Personality disorders include borderline personality disorder, antisocial personality disorder, and other similar illnesses. These disorders are defined by an "enduring pattern of inner experience and behavior that deviates markedly from the expectations of the culture of the individual who exhibits it" (APA, 2000, p. 686). The socially inappropriate patterns of behavior tend to be fixed and are present in all situations. The behavior is typically perceived to be appropriate by the individual, even when it results in negative outcomes in daily life (NIMH, 2010b). People with personality disorders are also very likely to have co-occurring major mental disorders, including anxiety disorders, mood disorders, impulse control disorders, and substance abuse or dependence (Lenzenweger, Lane, Loranger, & Kessler, 2007).

Sociocultural Influences

It is difficult to pinpoint the exact era of human history when mental health became a focus of inquiry and treatment (Bromberg, 1975). However, it is known that the identification of mental disorders was documented in the ancient world. The ancient Greeks classified mental illnesses not only according to outward symptoms and signs but also by acknowledging underlying physical causes. The word *melancholy* derives from the Greek word for black bile, which was believed to be the cause of prolonged sadness (Miller, 2010). The diagnosis and treatment of mental disorders has evolved to incorporate a more sophisticated understanding of these illnesses. Modern research in neuroscience and genetics has advanced the field to recognize the underlying biological contributors to mental illnesses. Harnessing this knowledge has improved the diagnosis and treatment of many disorders. NIMH (2010b) has recently instituted a new initiative to foster the research needed to create a new way of classifying mental disorders that is based on identifiable neural circuits. The current resource for classifying mental disorders in the United States is the *Diagnostic and Statistical Manual of Mental Disorders, Fourth Edition, Text Revision* (*DSM-IV-TR*).

In 1917, before the development of the first manual, the American Psychiatric Association (APA) and the New York Academy of Medicine collaborated to create a nationally recognized nomenclature for the classification of severe psychiatric and neurological disorders. During WWII, the U.S. Army developed a much broader nomenclature to address the needs of servicemen and veterans. At the same time, the WHO published the sixth edition of the *International Classification of Diseases* (*ICD-6*), which, for the first time, included a section for mental disorders. The *ICD-6* was greatly influenced by the Veterans Administration nomenclature, and the confluence of these attempts to classify mental disorders contributed to the first edition of the *Diagnostic and Statistical Manual of Mental Disorders* (*DSM-I*) in 1952. Since then, the manual has been amended and revised (APA, 2000). The fourth edition, the most current, represented a major advance in the diagnosis of mental disorders based in empirical research and relevant available data. Most diagnoses are founded on empirical literature. The current manual provides diagnostic criteria based on outward symptoms and, until research on the biological contributors to mental disorders becomes more advanced and exact, the *DSM* is the only nationally recognized resource available in the United States for classification and identification of these disorders. The fifth edition of it is to be released in May of 2013 to much anticipation in the mental health field, as the manual has not been revised since 2000. To track the advancement of the new edition, the APA has dedicated a part of its website to updates on the *DSM-V*'s progress (APA, 2010). Since the inception of the *DSM*, the identification of mental disorders has improved treatment outcomes and fostered the acknowledgment of mental disorders as a serious health issue that warrants attention.

Mental disorders are an immense psychological, social, and economic burden to society and increase the risk for physical illnesses. The WHO reports that about 450 million people suffer from mental and behavioral disorders worldwide and that 1 in 4 individuals will develop one or more of these disorders during their lifetime. Mental illnesses account for 13% of the total disability-adjusted life years (DALYs) lost due to all diseases and injuries in the world, and the number is estimated to increase to 15% by the year 2020. DALYs account for lost years of healthy life, regardless of whether the years were lost to premature death or disability. The disability component of the DALY measure is weighted by the severity of the disability. For example, major depressive disorder is considered the same in terms of burden as blindness or paraplegia whereas psychotic disorders, such as schizophrenia, are equal in disability burden to quadriplegia ("Mental Illness Overview," 2002). Out of the 10 leading causes of disability and premature death worldwide, 5 are related to mental disorders.

Depression is one of the most prevalent mental disorders, affecting approximately 340 million worldwide (WHO, 2004). By the year 2020, depression is expected to become the second-ranked cause of disease burden, accounting for 5.7% of DALYs, just behind ischemic heart disease. The anticipated increase of burden from depression means that one third of all worldwide disability will be from this one disorder, which has been identified as the most important mental disorder to address (WHO, 2004). Like depression, anxiety disorders are among the most prevalent mental disorders. Anxiety disorders affect about 40 million American adults ages 18 years and older (about 18% of this population) in a given year (Kessler, Chiu, Demler, & Walters, 2005). In terms of expense, anxiety disorders in the United States were estimated to have cost $64 billion dollars in 1990. In the past 50 years, eating disorders in developed countries have notably increased. Anorexia nervosa occurs in 0.5%-1.0% and bulimia nervosa in 0.9%-4.1% of the female adolescent and young adult population, while an additional 5.0%-13.0% suffer from partial syndrome eating disorders (APA, 2000). In the United States, anorexia nervosa is the third most common chronic condition in adolescent girls after obesity and asthma. The incidence and prevalence rates of eating disorders are low; however, the consequences of eating disorders contribute to an increased risk of a host of serious chronic disorders, like substance abuse, depression, and anxiety disorders, which contribute to a greater cost (NIMH, 2010b).

Bipolar disorder is a chronic mental illness that becomes a significant economic burden for those diagnosed, their families, and the larger society. For individuals aged 15-44 years worldwide, bipolar disorder is ranked 6th in the top 10 causes of disability (Murray & Lopez, 1996). Individuals with bipolar disorder often utilize social and welfare systems and require costly inpatient and outpatient treatment. Studies on the cost of bipolar disorder in the United States estimate expenditures at around $45.2 billion and $24 billion (Kleinman et al., 2003). Of the 2.6% of the U.S. population diagnosed with bipolar disorder, an estimated 82.9% are severe cases. Only about half (48.8%) of the individuals diagnosed are receiving treatment, and within that group, approximately 38.8% are receiving adequate treatment (Kessler, Burglund, et al., 2005; Kessler, Chiu, et al., 2005).

Psychotic disorders make up a small percentage of the mental health burden, but these disorders are most often severe and require multiple services. Schizophrenia is the most common psychotic illness and has a lifetime prevalence of approximately 1% with a point prevalence around .05%. Worldwide, schizophrenia was found to account for 2.8% of the years lost to death (YLD) and 1.1% of the DALYs (Murray et al., 2001). In comparison to other mental disorders, there are no major economic costs associated with schizophrenia; however, it is estimated to cost the United States around $19 billion in related services and provisions (WHO, 2010). Like schizophrenia, no major economic costs are associated with personality disorders; however, it is estimated that 39% of individuals with personality disorders seek treatment for other mental health issues, such as substance abuse and depression, and are more likely to receive treatment from general medical providers (Lenzenweger et al., 2007).

Cost-control efforts are evidenced in policy implementation such as the Patient Protection and Affordable Care Act (PPACA) of 2010, which set in motion the expansion of health insurance coverage and evaluation approaches to reduce health-care spending. In addition, mental health economic researchers meet regularly to discuss current spending issues in mental health. In 2011, the Biennial Research Conference on the Economics of Mental Health convened to focus on the challenges associated with health-care reform and mental health care financing. These efforts to control costs are informed by the 2008 Mental Health Parity and Addiction Equity Act, which requires that mental health benefits be equally covered with other medical benefits within an insurance plan. The challenge of cost-cutting decisions highlights the necessity of improving the quality of care and coverage of mental health.

The economic burden of mental disorders is recognized as a wide-ranging and long-lasting issue that imposes a range of costs on individuals, families, and communities. Increasingly, in the face of economic downturn, cost control is needed in all sectors of health care. In the United States, mental illness represents approximately 6% of overall health-care spending (Mark et al., 2007). Among all Americans, 36.2 million have paid for mental health services, totaling $57 billion in 2006 (Agency for Healthcare Research and Quality (AHRQ), 2006). These expenditures make mental disorders the third costliest medical conditions in the United States behind heart conditions and trauma and ties the disorders with cancer. The dollar amounts attached to mental health care only represent a fraction of the actual price of mental illness, which can result in other substantial costs for co-existing conditions and for society due to disability, unemployment, and incarceration (Insel, 2011).

Treatment

Recent research in drug treatments and psychotherapeutic interventions has brought relief to many individuals with mental illnesses. There has also been a resurgence of the use of brain stimulation therapies. The decision to seek treatment for a mental disorder can be difficult and finding the appropriate method(s) should involve the expert care of medical and mental health professionals. It is imperative to receive a correct diagnosis and to be monitored while receiving treatment to ensure the most positive outcome possible.

Medications are used to treat the symptoms of mental disorders, such as schizophrenia, depression, bipolar disorder, anxiety disorders, and attention deficit-hyperactivity disorder (ADHD), and can also be used in tandem with other treatments such as psychotherapy. Medication cannot cure a disorder. It can make people feel better so they are able to function. Some people experience positive results from medications and only need them for a short period. For example, an individual who suffers from depression may feel better after taking the medication for a few months and may never need it again. Individuals who have disorders such as anxiety, schizophrenia, or bipolar, long-term, or severe depression may need to take medication for a longer period, often for their whole lives. Some people experience side effects from medication. Factors such as dosage, type of mental disorder, age, sex, body size, physical illnesses, unhealthy habits such as smoking and drinking alcohol, liver and kidney function, genetics, and whether the medication is taken as prescribed affect how an individual responds to medication (NIMH, 2011).

Psychotherapy, or "talk therapy," is a method for treating mental disorders that assists individuals in understanding their illness and teaches them tools to manage symptoms and function optimally in everyday life. Psychotherapy alone has been proven effective for many with mental disorders. When that is not sufficient, it is often used in combination with medication. There are many types of psychotherapies, such as cognitive behavioral therapy, interpersonal therapy, family focused therapy, and a myriad of others to choose from based on personal and therapeutic needs. No "one-size-fits-all" psychotherapy exists, and some therapies have been scientifically studied more than others (NIMH, 2011).

Brain stimulation therapies, such as electroconvulsive therapy (ECT), involve activating or touching the brain directly with electricity, magnets, or implants to treat depression and other disorders. ECT, first developed in 1938, has the longest history of use and has been extensively researched compared to other newer, more experimental brain stimulation therapies, such as vagus nerve stimulation, repetitive transcranial magnetic stimulation, magnetic seizure therapy, and deep brain stimulation. ECT has been negatively depicted in popular culture for decades and had a poor reputation. It has been greatly improved and is now a safe and effective treatment option for individuals that do not respond to other treatments, such as medication or psychotherapy. It is most often used to treat severe treatment-resistant depression but has also been successful with other illnesses, such as bipolar disorder and schizophrenia (NIMH, 2011).

Complementary and alternative medicine (CAM) used as an adjunct or replacement of conventional medicine is on the rise in the United States (Perron, Jarman, & Kilbourne, 2009). Individuals with mental disorders have been found to be more likely to use CAM than those with other types of illnesses (Mamtani & Cimino, 2002). Although CAM treatments have limitations, many controlled studies have identified promising results in the areas of anxiety and depression. In addition, sufficient evidence supports the efficacy of treatments such as acupuncture for addiction problems and massage therapy and mind-body techniques like meditation, relaxation, and biofeedback for anxiety. Supplements like vitamins and herbal remedies are less understood and must be used with caution and under the care of a physician or psychiatrist (Mamtani & Cimino, 2002).

Prevention

Evidence-based policies and programs support the prevention of mental illness and cover the range of intervention modalities (primary, secondary, and tertiary). Interventions and research efforts tend to focus, for the major part, on risk factors (the negative influences on an individual's life that makes them more prone to mental disorders) and protective factors (those positive influences that reduce the likelihood an individual will develop a mental illness) involved in contributing to the onset of a mental illness. The development of a mental illness involves many risk and protective factors such as biology, family, psychology, environment, and social factors (WHO, 2004). Some prevention interventions have been found to reduce the onset of some disorders; however, more effective interventions need to be developed to address the current limitations in prevention of mental illnesses (WHO, 2004).

Due to the myriad of risk factors associated with mental disorders, prevention efforts target a wide range of issues. For example, some of the identified and targeted risk factors for the onset of depression include parental depression, inadequate parenting, child abuse, stressful events, and poverty. Protective factors like a sense of mastery, self-esteem, stress resistance, and social factors have also been identified as reducing the onset of depression. Anxiety disorders most often initially appear in childhood and adolescence, which makes these age groups a target for primary intervention. Populations at risk for anxiety disorders include children of anxious parents and victims of child abuse, accidents, violence, war, and other traumas. Adverse events in early childhood contribute to a neurological vulnerability that predisposes a child to anxiety disorders in adulthood. A vast body of research deals with eating disorders, but the onset of this disorder warrants increased attention to better inform prevention design. The current climate of eating disorders includes the identification of risk and protective factors such as peers, family, mass media, literacy, insecure attachment, physical and sexual abuse, low self-esteem, and difficulties coping healthfully with stress and conflict. Psychotic disorders, such as schizophrenia, have a complex etiology that is not well understood but known to involve major genetic contributions as well as environmental factors that interact with the genetic susceptibility (Jablensky & Kalaydjieva, 2003; van Os & McGuffin, 2003). Universal prevention is not yet possible for psychotic disorders as it is with other disorders such as communicable diseases that can be targeted through immunization or risk factors. Current efforts focus on encouraging those at risk to seek early help and developing improved methods for identifying individuals at risk for psychotic disorders (WHO, 2004).

Suicide is not considered a mental illness. It is a dire consequence of the lack of or inadequate identification and treatment of mental disorders. The WHO (2004) estimates that worldwide approximately 849,000 died from suicide in 2001, and this number is expected to increase to 1.2 million suicides in 2020 (Murray & Lopez, 1996). The most salient evidenced-based risk factors for suicide are mental disorders (mostly depression and schizophrenia), past or recent social stressors (e.g., childhood trauma, sexual or physical abuse, unemployment, social isolation, and serious economic problems), suicide in the family or peers, and low access to services of assistance. Planned attempts to reduce community rates of suicides have been implemented over the past decades, but the availability of evidence on the outcomes remains limited. To date, the most effective strategies to prevent suicides include the prescription of anti-depressant medications for individuals suffering from depression and the reduction of access to the means of committing suicide (e.g., removing firearms and medications). For youth, a multi-component school-based approach is recommended to emphasize prevention at an early age.

We interviewed Amanda, a 33-year-old woman, for her

experience with mental health issues. While in college, one of Amanda's friends committed suicide. Amanda's other friends became very concerned about the effect it had on Amanda and urged her to seek counseling. She went once and thought it was not for her. Amanda was in her early twenties the first time she consulted a therapist on her own. She believes she went due to an undesirable relationship. Since then, she has sought therapy on numerous occasions, seeing a therapist for periods of a year to a year and a half. After seeing her last therapist, she felt fine and therapy did not seem to be of use to her anymore. Amanda does believe she will probably continue to require therapy intermittently.

Amanda's mental health was in very poor condition about five years ago, and she began to suffer from insomnia then. Insomnia continues to plague her. She still depends on an over-the-counter sleep aid. Amanda took a break from school during that difficult time and began a relationship she now regrets. Her therapist at that time prescribed a medication for her depression and anxiety. Since then, Amanda has been prescribed several different medications, each one with side effects that have caused her to either switch to another medication or only take the medication from time to time. She has some readily available for when she needs to feel calm.

Others had told Amanda that, once she started taking medications, she was likely to have to take them her whole life and that scared her. She felt like she needed the medication to get her through the situation and that, if it improved, she would improve as well. It did get better for her so she has not taken medication regularly since. One doctor also told Amanda to quit drinking. Though she continues to drink now, a period of abstaining from alcohol made her realize the benefits of not medicating by drinking.

Amanda finds that one of the main difficulties in dealing with her mental health issue is concealing that she has a problem from other people. She also has trouble reconciling the despair and knowledge that her depression, though fleeting at times, will always be with her. Success has come for Amanda when she does not allow unfortunate situations in her life, including the trivial, to cause her extreme distress. Exercising and running frequently also facilitate the clearing of her mind and help stave off anxiety. She would recommend doing that and drinking less alcohol. She has also found that purposely spending a lot of time alone makes her want to be around other people more. She does not think anyone should force themselves to go out. Amanda does feel that she is now in a healthy relationship that significantly affirms her way of life. She also believes that working hard at her job and seeing tangible results makes her feel better about herself.

Amanda has a different perspective now and tries not to worry about the same things she did in her past. She is open to taking new medications for anxiety or depression, but she is limited to what her insurance covers and dealing with insurance is frustrating for her. Amanda believes she is fine now. At the time of the interview, she had not seen a therapist in almost a year.

To discover more about coping with a mental health issue, we interviewed Megan, a 33-year-old woman. Megan has bipolar disorder and suffers from major depression and manic episodes. She has been prescribed medication for each symptom. The greatest challenge Megan has had to face due to her disorder was deciding whether to have a child. Her mental health and the medication she was taking complicated the decision. She felt the common advice from obstetricians to stop all medications during pregnancy would not help in her situation. While pregnant, Megan felt the best she had ever felt and experienced a balance among her symptoms. She did fear depression would occur after the birth of her child and dreaded her bipolar disorder returning at that time.

Megan has not felt that she has failed in dealing with her disorder in a long time. In the past, she lapsed on taking her medication and drank instead. During those times, she would have awful relationships while her marriage disintegrated. She also did not sleep then and often thought of suicide. That was long ago for her. Megan believes that, if she stays on course, she will enjoy continued success.

Megan sees it fit to measure success in coping with her mental illness on her own scale. She believes a therapist, though valuable, cannot tell a person how to function in the world and with family. She finds her success is up to her, in her getting out of bed each day, taking care of her baby daughter, loving her family, and most importantly loving herself. For those coping with a mental health issue, Megan recommends ceasing the use of drugs and alcohol—other things capable of restraining a person's thoughts. She suggests finding a good therapist, someone trustworthy and respectful. And she suggests releasing the negativity and drama of the past, letting go of guilt and regrettable actions. Megan strongly advocates taking responsibility for one's own life, asking for help when needed, and forever loving oneself.

Conclusion

Tremendous strides in the diagnosis and treatment of mental disorders have been made over the last century and awareness of these illnesses continues to grow in the United States and throughout the world. The data related to mental illnesses underscores the urgency of treating and preventing mental disorders and promoting mental health as an important health issue. Much remains to be learned about the causes, treatment, and prevention of mental disorders. However, help and an array of well-documented treatments for mental disorders exist. Every person should be encouraged to seek help when faced with a mental illness just as they are encouraged to seek help for other health issues. Although disparities still exist in certain disadvantaged populations in the United States, many obstacles to effective treatment of mental disorders have been dismantled. Due to research and the study of the experiences of individuals who have a mental disorder and their family members and advocates, the efforts to battle mental illness have contributed to America's ability to respond to the needs of the mentally ill in an effective and respectful manner (U.S. Department of Health and Human Services, 1999).

Recommendations

A mental or behavioral disorder is characterized by a disturbance in thinking, mood, or behavior that is out of keeping with cultural beliefs and norms. In most cases the symptoms are associated with distress and interference with personal functions. Mental disorders produce symptoms that sufferers or those close to them notice. These may include:

- physical symptoms (e.g., aches and sleep disturbance)
- emotional symptoms (e.g., feeling sad, scared, or anxious)
- cognitive symptoms (e.g., difficulty thinking clearly, abnormal beliefs, and memory disturbance)
- behavioral symptoms (e.g., behaving in an aggressive manner, inability to perform routine daily functions, and excessive use of substances)
- perceptual symptoms (e.g. seeing or hearing things that others cannot)

Specific early signs vary from disorder to disorder. People who experience one or more of the symptoms listed above are encouraged to seek professional help if the symptoms persist, cause significant distress, or interfere with tasks of day-to-day living. In most cases mental disorders can be diagnosed and treated effectively (WHO, 2010).

Selected Resources

National Alliance on Mental Illness (NAMI)
3803 North Fairfax Drive, Suite 100
Arlington, VA 22203.
703-524-7600; Fax: 703-524-9094
www.nami.org/

National Institute of Mental Health (NIMH)
Science Writing, Press, and Dissemination Branch
6001 Executive Boulevard
Room 8184, MSC 9663

Bethesda, MD 20892-9663.
301-443-4513; 866-615-6464; TTY: 301-443-8431;
TTY toll-free: 866-415-8051;
Fax: 301-443-4279
nimhinfo@nih.gov
www.nimh.nih.gov/index.shtml

National Institutes of Health (NIH)
9000 Rockville Pike
Bethesda, MD 20892
301-496-4000; TTY: 301-402-9612
NIHinfo@od.nih.gov
health.nih.gov/category/MentalHealthandBehavior

**Substance Abuse and Mental Health Services
Administration (SAMHSA)**
SAMHSA's Health Information Network
P.O. Box 2345
Rockville, MD 20847-2345
240-276-1310; 240-276-1320
www.samhsa.gov/index.aspx

World Health Organization (WHO)
Avenue Appia 20
1211 Geneva 27
Switzerland
Phone: + 41 22 791 21 11; Fax: + 41 22 791 31 11
info@who.int
www.who.int/mental_health/en/

References

Agency for Healthcare Research and Quality (AHRQ). (2006). Studies highlight the value of the Medical Expenditure Panel Survey to inform trends in care costs, coverage, use, and access. *AHRQ Research Activities*, (312), 13-15.

American Psychiatric Association. (2000). *Diagnostic and statistical manual of mental disorders* (Revised 4th ed.). Washington, DC: Author.

American Psychiatric Association. (2010). DSM-5: The future of psychiatric diagnosis. Retrieved April 19, 2011, from http://www.dsm5.org/Pages/Default.aspx

Barber, C. (2008). The brain: A mindless obsession. *The Wilson Quarterly, 32*(1), 32-44.

Bromberg, W. (1975). *From shaman to psychotherapy: A history of the treatment of mental illness.* Chicago, IL: Regnery.

Herrman, H., Saxena, S., & Moodie, R. (Eds.). (2005). *Promoting mental health: Concepts, emerging evidence, practice. Report of the World Health Organization, Department of Mental Health and Substance Abuse in collaboration with the Victorian Health Promotion Foundation and the University of Melbourne.* Geneva, Switzerland: World Health Organization.

Insel, T. (2011, January 26). The economics of health care reform [Blog post]. Retrieved from http://www.nimh.nih.gov/about/director/2011/the-economics-of-health-care-reform.shtml

Jablensky, A., & Kalaydjieva, L. (2003). Genetic epidemiology of schizophrenia: Phenotypes, risk factors, and reproductive behavior. *American Journal of Psychiatry, 160*(3), 425-429.

Kessler, R. C., Berglund, P., Demler, O., Jin, R., Merikangas, K. R., & Walters, E. E. (2005). Lifetime prevalence and age-of-onset distributions of *DSM-IV* disorders in the National Comorbidity Survey Replication. *Archives of General Psychiatry, 62*(6), 593-602.

Kessler, R. C., Chiu, W. T., Demler, O., & Walters, E. E. (2005). Prevalence, severity, and comorbidity of twelve-month *DSM-IV* disorders in the National Comorbidity Survey Replication (NCS-R). *Archives of General Psychiatry, 62*(6), 617-627.

Kleinman, L., Lowin, A., Flood, E., Gandhi, G., Edgell, E., & Revicki, D. (2003). Costs of bipolar disorder. *Pharmacoeconomics, 21*, 601–622.

Lennox, B. R. (2009). The clinical experience and potential of brain imaging in patients with mental illness. *Frontiers in Human Neuroscience, 3*, 46.

Lenzenweger, M. F., Lane, M. C., Loranger, A. W., & Kessler, R. C. (2007). *DSM-IV* personality disorders in the National Comorbidity Survey Replication. *Biological Psychiatry, 62*(6), 553-564.

Mamtani, R., & Cimino, A. (2002). A primer of complementary and alternative medicine and its relevance in the treatment of mental health problems. *Psychiatric Quarterly, 73*(4), 367-381.

Mark, T. L., Levit, K. R., Coffey, R. M., McKusick, D. R., Harwood, H. J., King, E. C., . . . Ryan, K. (2007). *National expenditures for mental health services and substance abuse treatment, 1993-2003* (SAMHSA Publication No. SMA 07-4227). Retrieved from http://www.samhsa.gov/spendingestimates/SAMHSAFINAL9303.pdf

Mental illness overview. (2002). *Congressional Digest, 81*(1), 1-3.

Miller, G. (2010). Beyond *DSM*: Seeking a brain-based classification of mental illness. *Science, 327*(5972), 1437.

Murray, C. J., & Lopez, A. D. (Eds.). (1996). *The global burden of disease: A comprehensive assessment of mortality and disability from diseases, injuries and risk factors in 1990 and projected to 2020.* Cambridge, MA: Harvard University Press.

Murray C.J. et al. (2001). *The global burden of disease 2000 project: aims, methods, and data sources.* Geneva, World Heath Organization.

National Alliance on Mental Illness. (n.d.). Mental illnesses. Retrieved April 11, 2011, from http://www.nami.org/Content/NavigationMenu/Inform_Yourself/About_Mental_Illness/About_Mental_Illness.htm

National Institute of Mental Health. (n.d.). The science of mental illness: Information about mental illness and the brain. Retrieved April 11, 2011, from http://science.education.nih.gov/supplements/nih5/mental/guide/info-mental-a.htm

National Institute of Mental Health. (2010a). Any disorder among adults. Retrieved April 11, 2011, from http://www.nimh.nih.gov/statistics/1ANYDIS_ADULT.shtml

National Institute of Mental Health. (2010b). *From discovery to cure: Accelerating the development of new and personalized interventions for mental illnesses. Report of the National Advisory Mental Health Council's Workgroup.* Retrieved from http://www.nimh.nih.gov/about/advisory-boards-and-groups/namhc/reports/fromdiscoverytocure.pdf

National Institute of Mental Health. (2011). Health topics. Retrieved

April 11, 2011, from http://www.nimh.nih.gov/health/index. shtml

Perron, B. E., Jarman, C. N., & Kilbourne, A. M. (2009). Access to conventional mental health and medical care among users of complementary and alternative medicine with bipolar disorder. *The Journal of Nervous and Mental Disease, 197*(4), 287-290.

U.S. Department of Health and Human Services. (1999). *Mental health: A report of the Surgeon General.* Rockville, MD: Author.

U.S. Department of Health and Human Services, National Institutes of Health, National Institute of Mental Health. (n.d). *Neuroimaging and mental illness: A window into the brain* (NIH Publication No. 09-7460). Bethesda, MD: Author.

van Os, J., & McGuffin, P. (2003). Can the social environment cause schizophrenia? *British Journal of Psychiatry, 182*(4), 291-292.

World Health Organization. (2004). *Prevention of mental disorders: Effective interventions and policy options. Summary report: A report of the World Health Organization Department of Mental Health and Substance Abuse in collaboration with the Prevention Research Centre of the Universities of Nijmegen and Maastricht.* Geneva, Switzerland: Author.

World Health Organization. (2010). Mental health: Strengthening our response (Fact sheet No. 220). Retrieved from http//www. who.int/mediacentre/factsheets/fs220/en/index.html

SPIRITUALITY
AND HEALTH

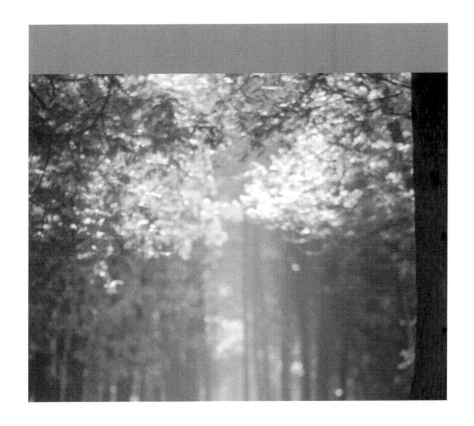

More individuals in the United States than in any other industrialized country identify personal spiritual and religious beliefs, practices, and affiliations as a major component of their lives (Christiano, Swatos, & Kivisto, 2002; Gallup & Lindsay, 1999; Kosmin & Lachman, 1993; Spilka, Hood, Hunsberger, & Gorusch, 2003). The practice of religion and spirituality has remained a major influence on American public and private life since the beginning of the Colonial Period. This practice and health have long had a tumultuous and complex relationship. At times throughout world history, religion and health were synonymous: medicine and pious practice were performed by the same person. At other times, they have been in stark contrast, medicine becoming a separate, distinct field from religion.

In recent decades, health research has reflected attempts to explore a more symbiotic relationship between medicine and spirituality in order to optimize health outcomes for individuals. Some studies have found an association between spiritual and religious affiliation and increased health and wellness whereas other studies have found that the affiliation can have a negative effect or none at all (Ferraro & Kelley-Moore, 2000). Although religion has for hundreds of years contributed to America's cultural landscape, it has increasingly become more fluid and adaptable, represented by a variety of related practices (Gallup Poll, 2010). Religious trends have moved in a new direction, one representing a more ecumenical and flexible conceptualization of religion. More Americans may not be affiliating themselves with a specific religious tradition, but this does not mean they are without a spiritual identity (Bader et al., 2006).

Spirituality Versus Religiosity

In recent decades, a shift has occurred from using the term *religion* to the more inclusive, and yet more vague, concept of *spirituality* (Hatch, Burg, Naberhaus, & Hellmich, 1998; Underwood & Teresi, 2002), reflecting the notion that religion is tied to the historical and dogmatic baggage of many faiths and is less desirable to represent an individual's beliefs. Spirituality is often viewed as a more ecumenical and encompassing mode of expressing belief in something larger than oneself. The differentiation between religiosity and spirituality remains somewhat contentious and not well defined across disciplines (Hatch et al., 1998; Underwood & Teresi, 2002). This can make it difficult to conduct research and determine how to define the aspect of religion or spirituality that is being measured. However, over the past 35 years, studies using the term *spirituality* and health have increased, while there has been a decrease in studies using the term *religion* and health, indicating that *spirituality* is becoming the preferred term (Chiu, Emblen, Van Hofwegen, Sawatzky, & Meyerhoff, 2004). It is common to see both terms used interchangeably at times and at other times in stark contrast in related health literature. *Spirituality* and its related words will be used in the rest of this chapter to reduce confusion and to represent the current trend in term usage.

Sociocultural Influences

The scientific study of spirituality traces back to the end of the 19th century and the beginning of the 20th century, when books were published by social philosophers William James and Max Weber, which contributed to the development of recognized fields of study in the psychology and sociology of spirituality. The 1920s and 1930s saw a rejection of the study of spirituality and a rise in the disciplines of behaviorism, psychoanalysis, and related areas of study. But rumblings of studies and attention regarding spirituality and health still lingered in the face of intellectual and scientific predominance and were influential on subsequent generations of research (Cockerham, 2010).

Although spirituality and health have been entwined for eons, literature regarding the health impact of spirituality and integration of it into health practices originated in the late 20th century (Mills, 2002; Seybold, 2007). The first tools of measurement to determine the relationship between spirituality and health were developed after WWII (Allport, 1950; Allport & Ross, 1967; Glock & Stark, 1966; Hood, 1975; King & Hunt, 1967). One of the main issues with these early developments was that they were greatly influenced by culture and assumptions that spirituality was either irrelevant (Rozin, 2001) or even pathological (Seybold, 2007). In the 1970s, less research was conducted in the area of spirituality and health, possibly due to the secular shift in American culture (Hall, Meador, & Koenig, 2008). Research resurged in the 1980s and 1990s, introducing a more open approach to studying the relationship between spirituality and health (Emmons & Paloutzian, 2003; Gorsuch, 1984; Gorsuch & McPherson, 1989; Larson, Swyers, & McCullough, 1997; Levin, 1994; Koenig, Parkerson, & Meador, 1997; Pargament, 1997), including a more nuanced and salutogenic focus, such as on forgiveness and positive coping.

Since the resurgence of the 1980s and 1990s, movement has increased in the health field to recognize spirituality as a salient aspect of overall health (Lee & Newberg, 2005). In recent years, most every health-related journal has included articles on the relationship between spirituality and health (Mills, 2002). This reasonably new phenomena has been attributed to factors such as the rise in use of complementary and holistic health practices and the more impersonal philosophy of managed care that has spurred patients to demand acknowledgment of other modalities of health care that can be used in conjunction with Western medical practices (Cangialose, Cary, Hoffman, & Ballard, 1997; Lee & Newberg, 2005; Mills, 2002). Ample evidence also indicates that the role of spirituality in health care is increasing and that health-care workers are more apt to acknowledge the importance of this role in providing services (Chiu et al., 2004). Several prominent organizations have recognized the importance of spirituality in health care. The Joint Commission on Accreditation of Healthcare Organizations (1999) implemented policy stating that "for many patients, pastoral care and other spiritual services are an integral part of health care and daily life. The hospital is able to provide for pastoral care and other spiritual services for patients who request them" (p. xxx). The American College of Physicians created a panel to discuss end-of-life care and the need for doctors to pay attention to providing for psychosocial, existential, or spiritual suffering (Lo, Quill, & Tulsky, 1999).

Biology and Physiology

William James (1902), in his seminal work *The Varieties of Religious Experience*, addresses the lack of scientific study on the physiological effects of spiritual practice by stating that "some psychophysical theory connecting spiritual values in general with determinate sorts of physiological change" must be identified to treat the overall health of individuals (p. 16). Although this suggestion was made over a century ago now, minimal research on the biological and physiological components of spiritual practice has been done. Attempting to measure the biological impact of spirituality has proven to be daunting in multiple ways. Many studies of this nature experience problems related to research methods, which make determining a direct causal relationship difficult (Koenig & Cohen, 2002). Spirituality is comprised of features that can be representative of factors that are not necessarily spiritual. Spirituality is a more esoteric concept compared to other health issues such as nutrition and physical activity, which are measurable and observable. It is challenging to distill the essence of spirituality and determine what it is about spirituality that contributes to health outcomes.

The limited research conducted on the topic of spirituality and health is especially apparent in the amount of research on the Judeo-Christian tradition. The majority of studies conducted to measure the health-related biological responses to Judeo-Christian spiritual practice consist of only three different propositions: (1) spirituality is associated with lower blood pressure and less hypertension; (2) spirituality is associated with better lipid profiles (i.e., lower LDL and higher HDL cholesterol); and (3) spirituality is associated with better immune function (Seeman, Dubin, & Seeman, 2003).

Studies examining lower blood pressure and hypertension generally show a significant relationship with church attendance (Graham et al., 1978; Hixson, Gruchow, & Morgan, 1998; Koenig et al., 1997; Larson, Swyers, & McCullough, 1998; Livingston, Levine, & Moore, 1991; Scotch, 1963), spiritual commitment (Hixson et al., 1998; Steffen, Hinderliter, Blumenthal, & Sherwood, 2001; Walsh, 1998), and being a nun in comparison to being a laywoman (Timio et al., 1997). Studies comparing Orthodox Jews and secular individuals observed differences in lipid profiles between the two groups (Friedlander, Kark, Kaufmann, & Stein, 1985; Friedlander, Kark, & Stein, 1987). The groups of Orthodox Jews in both studies were found to have lower total cholesterol, LDL cholesterol ("bad" cholesterol), and triglyceride levels. Triglyceride is the form that most fat takes in the body. If triglyceride levels are too high, it can contribute to heart disease, stroke, diabetes, and other related illnesses. Problematically, diet was not controlled for and may have been the biggest contributing factor to the lowered triglyceride and cholesterol levels (Seeman et al., 2003).

Studies on immune function have shown some promise. One study (Koenig et al., 1997) examining church attendance and various biological elements of immune function revealed a significant association between church attendance and lower levels of Interleukin-6, a marker of inflammation related to antibody production and immune function, within the cross-sectional data but not the longitudinal data. Other markers of immune function, like alpha-1, alpha-2, beta globulin, gamma gobulin, lymphocytes, and D-dimer, were not related significantly in any way to church attendance. Another study (Woods, Antoni, Ironson, & Kling, 1999) examined prayer and spiritual service attendance and T helper/inducer cell (CD4+) counts and percentages in HIV-positive gay males. CD4+ works with other lymphocytes (either T or B) to initiate immune functions. Findings from the study supported the hypothesis that spiritual behavior accounted for higher CD4+ counts and percentages, indicating a relationship between spirituality and increased immune function. Other studies examining spiritual behavior and immune function found a significant relationship between spirituality and lower cortisol (a hormone released by the adrenal gland when a person is under stress) levels in individuals (Ironson et al., 2002; Sephton, Sapolsky, Kraemer, & Spiegel, 2000) and higher white blood cells (indicating stronger immune function) in breast cancer patients (Sephton, Koopman, Schaal, Thoresen, & Spiegel, 2001). As technology and science combine to expand current methods of gathering knowledge and testing physiological associations with spirituality, researchers will use more sophisticated and multi-faceted assessments to include multiple biological systems instead of singular measurements, such as blood pressure and cortisol levels (Seeman et al., 2003).

Compared to studies on Judeo-Christianity and health, practices such as meditation and yoga have been studied more in depth and benefit from a much larger array of research measuring physiological impact. Although meditation and yoga are most often associated with Eastern spiritual traditions, not all of the studies discussed here explicitly stated a spiritual affiliation in their reports. Meditation and yoga are techniques that can be practiced and adapted outside of their spiritual affiliations. However, these techniques represent a component of spiritual practice and originate from spiritual traditions and therefore continue to be included in health and spiritual literature.

A three-month intensive yoga training program was implemented with an experimental group of participants, and physiological outcomes were compared with a control group of age- and gender-matched participants. Yoga participants exhibited reductions in cholesterol, blood pressure, fibrinogen (a protein needed for blood coagulation), and body mass compared to the control group. However, the experimental group showed an increase in cortisol, which may have been due to group differences that were not factored into the analyses (Schmidt, Wijga, Von Zur Muhlen, Brabant, & Wagner, 1997). A group of patients with carpal-tunnel syndrome volunteered for an eight-week yoga-based program and reported improved grip strength and reductions in pain at the end of the intervention (Garfinkel et al., 1998).

Other studies have examined the effects of meditation training and relaxation techniques on patients with differing ailments. In the 1970s, researchers began studying brain activity in relation to meditation practices and/or biofeedback. Biofeedback is a process by which individuals apply cognitive control techniques, like visualization and relaxation, and can be used for a number of disorders and physiological responses (American Psychiatric Association Task Force on Biofeedback, 1980; Barber et al., 1971; Hirai, 1974; Marcer, 1986). These early studies suggested that meditation could result in lower levels of physiological responses through the mediation of the brain. For example, one study examined the electroencephalogram (EEG) of volunteers participating in a program implementing relaxation techniques. The findings revealed a reduction in frontal EEG beta activity, which indicates a lowered stress response. Changes in body metabolism and an *increase* in beta activity were observed in a study of Tibetan Buddhist monks practicing meditation, indicating that it is possible that different types of meditative practice may have different effects on practitioners (Benson, Malhotra, Goldman, Jacobs, & Hopkins, 1990).

The body of research focusing on the effects of meditation/relaxation-related interventions in clinical populations has been growing (Seeman et al., 2003). Kabat-Zinn and colleagues (1992, 1998) developed a meditation-based stress reduction program employing mindfulness meditation, or "paying attention in a particular way: on purpose, in the present moment, and nonjudgmentally" (Kabat-Zinn, 1994, p. 4). Mindfulness meditation entails multiple areas of concentration (like breath and body awareness), distinguishing it from transcendental meditation, which requires the repetition of a mantra to enhance focus and relaxation. Mindfulness meditation interventions resulted in reductions in anxiety and depression in patients with generalized anxiety or panic disorders (Kabat-Zinn et al., 1992), and for patients with psoriasis, clearing up of the condition was quicker (Kabat-Zinn et al., 1998).

Mandle et al. (1990) recruited patients undergoing femoral artery angiographies and found that the group assigned to listen to a relaxation audiotape reported less anxiety and pain than those with music or a blank audiotape; however, no physiological responses, such as with blood pressure or heart rate, were found. Other older studies on the effectiveness of meditation/yoga interventions for reducing blood pressure among those who have hypertension showed mixed results, some reporting a reduction (Patel & North, 1975; Sundar et al., 1984) and other studies not (Hafner, 1982; Pollack, Case, Weber, & Laragh, 1977).

Some studies have examined cardiovascular function (blood pressure and cholesterol), oxidative stress and stress hormones, and patterns of brain activity in relation to meditation. One randomized, longitudinal study observed subjects who had major risk factors for cardiovascular disease and measured the impact of an eight-week meditation/relaxation intervention on two or all of the risk factors (smoking, blood pressure, and cholesterol). The subjects in the meditation/relaxation group showed a significant decrease in blood pressure at eight weeks, eight months, and four years post-intervention and lower cholesterol levels at eight weeks and eight months post-intervention. When checked at four years post-intervention, those in the control group showed greater vulnerability to heart attack and greater incidence of cardiac events (Patel et al., 1985).

Another study (Schneider et al., 1995) examined the effects of a three-month program of transcendental meditation (TM) on the reduction of blood pressure in a sample of mildly hypertensive African American adults aged 55 and older. Subjects in the experimental group had significantly reduced blood pressure, and TM was found to be twice as effective as the control interventions.

Cortisol activity was measured in a group of novice practitioners of TM and compared to a control group of long-term practitioners of TM (Jevning, Wilson, & Davidson, 1978). Findings revealed that the long-term practitioners had the lowest levels of cortisol and that the novice group, when assessed a second time during the intervention, had cortisol values midway between their initial (pre-intervention) assessment and those of the long-term practitioners. The pattern indicates that long-term practice may have more salutary effects than short-term interventions (Jevning et al., 1978).

A three-year longitudinal study on male TM practitioners reported an increase of immune function but no change in stress response (Werner et al., 1986). Schneider et al. (1998) used a cross-sectional design to compare long-term TM practitioners with non-practitioners by using lipid peroxide levels as a marker for group differences in oxidative stress. Both lipid peroxide and oxidative stress are related to cell death and production of free radicals. The TM practitioners had lower levels of serum lipid peroxides than the control group of non-practitioners. In spite of potential confounding due to group differences and other factors, these studies fall in line with other research showing that TM contributes to lower physiological stress indicators (Infante et al., 1998; MacLean et al., 1997; Walton, Pugh, Gelderloos, & Macrae, 1995).

A range of physiological parameters were measured in a group of Thai college students who volunteered to participate in a two-month program of meditation training. The study also utilized a control group of Thai students who did not participate in any type of intervention. At the end of the two months, the meditation group displayed greater decreases in cortisol, systolic and diastolic blood pressure, and pulse rate than the control group (Sudsang, Chentanez, & Veluvan, 1991).

Prevention and Treatment

The multiple behaviors, attitudes, and beliefs that comprise spiritual practice have been shown to contribute to varied health outcomes. Spirituality is unlike the more researched and recognized health behaviors such as exercise and diet. It is well known that meeting the recommended requirements for exercise and diet can prevent chronic diseases and comprise treatment plans for illnesses such as diabetes and heart disease. No direct links between spirituality and the prevention or treatment of certain illnesses exist; however, relationships have been detected between certain health outcomes and behaviors related to spiritual practice. Spiritual practice can provide social support, dietary guidelines, life purpose, reassurance in stressful life situations, coping strategies, and other factors that are associated with positive health outcomes.

Attendance at spiritual services and prayers are two types of behavior in particular that have been researched intensively. Frequency of spiritual service attendance has been linked with reduced mortality (Strawbridge, Shema, Cohen, & Kaplan, 2001) and increased psychological well-being (Ellison, 1991). Prayer has been shown to be associated with positive health outcomes when used as a coping strategy (Shaw et al., 2007) and has also been associated with well-being in non-clinical populations (Maltby, Lewis, & Day, 1999). In addition, factors such as intrinsic spirituality (an internal motivation for spiritual behavior) have been connected with increased well-being in several studies (Byrd, Hageman, & Belle Isle, 2007; Maltby & Day, 2003). Having experiences perceived as sacred has also been found to be related to psychological health (Byrd, Lear, & Schwenka, 2000; Goldstein, 2007) and overall physical health (Koenig, George, & Titus, 2004). Some evidence indicates that individuals who, in particular, have spiritual beliefs and experiences that are positively framed benefit from spiritual practice (Byrd et al., 2000). Another aspect of spiritual behavior is the capacity for spirituality to provide a sense of existential certainty that may be an important contributing factor to overall well-being (Ellison, 1991).

Spiritual practice is often associated with a community of others that share the same or similar beliefs. Ample research has focused on the social aspects of spiritual practice and has revealed that spiritual group members provide other members with social support, such as material assistance and emotional support, through formal and informal channels. Some studies argue that the social component of spiritual practice is one of the main contributors to the positive health outcomes that individuals have experienced (Hayward & Elliot, 2009). Well-being has been linked to the amount of social support one receives and having a sense of involvement in the spiritual group (Greenfield & Marks, 2007; Koenig & Larson, 2001). However, studies have also shown that social involvement with spiritual groups can also have negative effects on well-being if individuals in the group are perceived as being critical or demanding (Krause, Ellison, & Wulff, 1999) or when conflict arises between members (Krause, Chatters, Meltzer, & Morgan, 2000).

The health outcomes of spirituality have also been found to be influenced by demographic predictors of well-being. Typically, certain demographic groups experience superior overall psychological and physiological health, such as youth (Mirowsky & Ross, 1992), men (Piccinelli & Wilkinson, 2000), people who are married (Mookherjee, 1997), members of racial and ethnic majority groups (Kutner, Bliwise, & Zhang, 2004), individuals who have received more education (Ross & Van Willigen, 1997), and those with higher incomes (Diener & Biswas-Diener, 2002). Due to the privileged health status of these groups, spirituality may have less impact on their health outcomes than on other less privileged groups. Research suggests that spiritual factors actually have the most positive impact on health outcomes within disadvantaged populations. For example, one study (Krause, 1998) found that spirituality was only associated with reduced mortality for older adults with low levels of education. Banthia, Moskowitz, Acree, and Folkman (2007) reported that higher frequency of prayer only increases positive self-assessed health outcomes in individuals with low education levels. These results suggest that spirituality can function as a buffering effect against lower socioeconomic status (Hayward & Elliott, 2009) or possibly that highly educated people tend to be less likely to derive a sense of life purpose from their spirituality (Stark, 2001).

For further insight into how spirituality can affect one's health, we interviewed Audrey, a 28-year-old woman. Audrey has accepted the Lord as her personal savior and professes a strong relationship with Him. She regularly prays and does so when she or her loved ones endure health problems. Audrey has faith in His will and recognizes that it may mean that not everyone will be healed. Though she had prayed for her, Audrey lost her grandmother to liver cancer. Audrey was grateful to Him for not allowing her grandmother to suffer and for helping her deal with the loss. Audrey notes that her grandmother was saved by His grace about five years ago, and Audrey has faith that she will meet her grandmother again in Heaven. This belief allows Audrey to continue on through each day.

One of the greatest difficulties Audrey has in her experience with spirituality and health is dealing with people that possess no faith in the Lord. Due to their lack of faith, she has trouble comforting them if they are suffering from a health issue. Though she may still speak of the Lord to those who do not believe, it is very challenging. She cannot relate to them. Audrey's customary advice to those who do believe is to pray to God for healing and, if it is not in His will to heal, to pray for His grace and comfort through the ordeal. Audrey believes there is hope with Him and, without Him, no hope.

Audrey's approach to spirituality—her prayer and placing all her faith in God—allows her to see "success" in every situation. She has only felt that she has failed when she is disobedient to the Lord. Audrey does experience times of doubt, fear, and worry. Those moments are not because she is thinking about death. She knows she is going to Heaven. Audrey believes in His will, good or bad, and surrenders herself to it. It is her confidence in His plan that gives her solace. For those using spirituality to cope with a health issue, she suggests giving themselves fully to God and trusting Him in his supreme power and knowledge. Audrey believes in a reliance on Him and only Him to survive through health issues.

To learn how spirituality can affect a person's health and well-being, we interviewed Michelle, a 34-year-old woman. Michelle considers herself a very spiritual person. When she has dealt with a health issue, she has used prayer to bring herself peace. Michelle often combines physician guidance with spiritual guidance to ensure she takes her medication regularly or to instruct her on how to engage in healing behaviors both outside and in.

For example, Michelle has found success in the "insight" she has received to get more rest and take part in stress-relieving activities. Though spiritual activities, such as prayer and scripture reading, benefit Michelle's well-being, she does find it challenging to regularly perform them. But, for those using spirituality to cope with a health issue, Michelle does recommend praying and having the faith that God or another higher power will provide guidance and bring peace.

Conclusion

Although a significant shift in spiritual affiliation has occurred in the United States, the majority of Americans continue to identify spirituality as a very important component of their lives. In recent decades, the demand for therapeutic practices that acknowledge and even incorporate personal spiritual beliefs has grown. Research in this area has increased to address the need for evidence-based studies on the health benefits and disadvantages of spirituality. It is difficult to make definite conclusions about the salutary effects of spiritual beliefs and practice because many of the contributors to increased health associated with spirituality are also identifiable outside the realm of spiritual practice. However, evidence supports the notion that aspects of spirituality assist individuals with issues such as hypertension, coping with illness, and stress, and spirituality has also been associated with reduced mortality.

Recommendations

One's spirituality is a very personal decision and no official recommendations from any entity in the health field exist. Those who wish for more information can consult the reference page and selected resources.

Selected Resources

FamilyDoctor.org
familydoctor.org/online/famdocen/home/articles/650.html

Healthy.net
www.healthy.net/scr/mainlinks.aspx?id=295

Journal of Religion and Health
Springer
233 Spring Street
New York, NY 10013
212-460-1500; 800-SPRINGER; Fax: 212-460-1575
service-ny@springer.com
www.springer.com/public+health/journal/10943

References

Allport, G. (1950). *The individual and his religion: A psychological interpretation.* New York: Macmillan.

Allport, G., & Ross, J. (1967). Personal religious orientation and prejudice. *Journal of Personality and Social Psychology, 5,* 447-457.

American Psychiatric Association Task Force on Biofeedback. (1980). *Biofeedback: Report of the Task Force on Biofeedback of the American Psychiatric Association* (Task Force Report No. 19). Washington, DC: American Psychiatric Association.

Bader, C., Dougherty, K., Froese, P., Johnson, B., Mencken, F. C., Park, J. Z., & Stark, R. (2006). *American piety in the 21st century: New insights to the depth and complexity of religion in the US - Selected findings from The Baylor Religion Survey.* Waco, TX: Baylor Institute for Studies of Religion.

Banthia, R., Moskowitz, J. T., Acree, M., & Folkman, S. (2007). Socioeconomic differences in the effects of prayer on physical symptoms and quality of life. *Journal of Health Psychology, 12,* 249-260.

Barber, T., DiCara, L. V., Kamiya, J., Miller, N. E., Shapiro, D., & Stoyva, J. (Eds.). (1971). *Biofeedback and self-control: An Aldine reader on the regulation of bodily processes and consciousness.* Chicago, IL: Aldine-Atherton.

Benson, H., Malhotra, M. S., Goldman, R. F., Jacobs, G. D., & Hopkins, J. (1990). Three case reports of the metabolic and electroencephalographic changes during advanced Buddhist meditation techniques. *Behavioral Medicine, 16,* 90-95.

Byrd, K. R., Hageman, A., & Belle Isle, D. (2007). Intrinsic motivation and subjective well-being: The unique contribution of intrinsic religious motivation. *International Journal for the Psychology of Religion, 17*(2), 141-156.

Byrd, K. R., Lear, D., & Schwenka, S. (2000). Mysticism as a predictor of subjective well-being. *International Journal for the Psychology of Religion, 10*, 259-270.

Cangialose, C. B., Cary, S. J., Hoffman, L. H., & Ballard, D. J. (1997). Impact of managed care on quality of healthcare: Theory and evidence. *American Journal of Managed Care, 3*, 1153-1170.

Chiu, L., Emblen, J. D., Van Hofwegen, L., Sawatzky, R., & Meyerhoff, H. (2004). An integrative review of the concept of spirituality in the health sciences. *Western Journal of Nursing Research, 26*(4), 405-428.

Christiano, K. J., Swatos, W. H., Jr., & Kivisto, P. (2002). *Sociology of religion: Contemporary developments.* Walnut Creek, CA: AltaMira Press.

Cockerham, W. C. (Ed.). (2010). *The new Blackwell companion to medical sociology.* Oxford, England: Wiley-Blackwell.

Diener, E., & Biswas-Diener, R. (2002). Will money increase subjective well-being? *Social Indicators Research, 57*, 119-169.

Ellison, C. G. (1991). Religious involvement and subjective well-being. *Journal of Health and Social Behavior, 32*(1), 80-99.

Emmons, R. A., & Paloutzian, R. F. (2003). The psychology of religion. *Annual Review of Psychology, 54*, 377-402.

Ferraro, K. F., & Kelley-Moore, J. A. (2000). Religious consolation among men and women: Do health problems spur seeking? *Journal for the Scientific Study of Religion, 39*(2), 220-234.

Friedlander, Y., Kark, J. D., Kaufmann, N., & Stein, Y. (1985). Coronary heart disease risk factors among religious groupings in a Jewish population sample in Jerusalem. *The American Journal of Clinical Nutrition, 42*(3), 511-521.

Friedlander, Y., Kark, J. D., & Stein, Y. (1987). Religious observance and plasma lipids and lipoproteins among 17-year-old Jewish residents of Jerusalem. *Preventive Medicine, 16*, 70-79.

Gallup, G., Jr., & Lindsay, D. M. (1999). *Surveying the religious landscape: Trends in US beliefs*. Harrisburg, PA: Morehouse.

Gallup. (2010). Religion [Webpage]. Retrieved April 19, 2011, from http://www.gallup.com/poll/1690/Religion.aspx#1

Garfinkel, M. S., Singhal, A., Katz, W. A., Allan, D. A., Reshetar, R., & Schumacher, H. R., Jr. (1998). Yoga-based intervention for carpal tunnel syndrome: A randomized trial. *Journal of the American Medical Association, 280*(18), 1601-1603.

Glock, C., & Stark, R. (1966). *Christian beliefs and anti-Semitism*. New York, NY: Harper & Row.

Goldstein, E. D. (2007). Sacred moments: Implications on well-being and stress. *Journal of Clinical Psychology, 63*, 1001-1019.

Gorsuch, R. (1984). Measurement: The boon and bane of investigating religion. *American Psychologist, 39*, 228-236.

Gorsuch, R., & McPherson, S. (1989). Intrinsic/extrinsic measurement: I/E—revised and single-item scales. *Journal for the Scientific Study of Religion, 28*, 348-354.

Graham, T. W., Kaplan, B. H., Cornoni-Huntley, J. C., James, S. A. Q., Becker, C., Hames,

C. G., & Heyden, S. (1978). Frequency of church attendance and blood pressure elevation. *Journal of Behavioral Medicine, 1,* 37-43.

Greenfield, E. A., & Marks, N. F. (2007). Religious social identity as an explanatory factor for associations between more frequent formal religious participation and psychological well-being. *International Journal for the Psychology of Religion, 17,* 245-259.

Hafner, R. J. (1982). Psychological treatment of essential hypertension: A controlled comparison of meditation and meditation plus biofeedback. *Biofeedback and Self Regulation, 7,* 305-316.

Hall, D. E., Meador, K. G., & Koenig, H. G. (2008). Measuring religiousness in health research: Review and critique. *Journal of Religion & Health, 47*(2), 134-163.

Hatch, R. L., Burg, M. A., Naberhaus, D. S., & Hellmich, L. K. (1998). The spiritual involvement and beliefs scale: Development and testing of a new instrument. *Journal of Family Practice, 46,* 476-486.

Hayward, R. D., & Elliott, M. (2009). Fitting in with the flock: Social attractiveness as a mechanism for well-being in religious groups. *European Journal of Social Psychology, 39*(4), 592-607.

Hirai, T. (1974). *Psychophysiology of Zen.* Tokyo, Japan: Igaku Shoin.

Hixson, K. A., Gruchow, H. W., & Morgan, D. W. (1998). The relation between religiosity, selected health behaviors, and blood pressure among adult females. *Preventive Medicine, 27,* 545-552.

Hood, R., Jr. (1975). The construction and preliminary validation of a measure of reported mystical experience. *Journal for the Scientific Study of Religion, 14*, 29-41.

Infante, J. R., Peran, F., Martinez, M., Roldan, A., Poyatos, R., Ruiz, C., . . . Garrido, F. (1998). ACTH and beta-endorphin in transcendental meditation. *Physiology & Behavior, 64*(3), 311-315.

Ironson, G., Solomon, G. F., Balbin, E. G., O'Cleirigh, C., George, M. A., Kumar, M., . . . Woods, T. E. (2002). The Ironson-Woods Spirituality/Religiousness Index is associated with long survival, health behaviors, less distress, and low cortisol in people with HIV/AIDS. *Annals of Behavioral Medicine, 24*, 34-48.

James, W. (1961). *The varieties of religious experience: A study in human nature.* Cambridge, MA: Harvard University Press. (Original work published 1902).

Jevning, R., Wilson, A. F., & Davidson, J. M. (1978). Adrenocorticol activity during meditation. *Hormones and Behavior, 10*(1), 54-60.

Joint Commission on Accreditation of Healthcare Organizations. (1999). Patient rights and organization ethics. In *Comprehensive accreditation manual for hospitals (CAMH): The official handbook* (Update 3, pp. R1-15.). Oakbrook Terrace, IL: Author.

Kabat-Zinn, J., Massion, A. O., Kristeller, J., Peterson, L. G., Fletcher, K. E., Pbert, L., . . . Santorelli, S. F. (1992). Effectiveness of a meditation-based stress reduction program in the treatment of anxiety disorders. *American Journal of Psychiatry, 149*(7), 936-943.

Kabat-Zinn, J. (1994). *Wherever you go, there you are.* New York: Hyperion.

Kabat-Zinn, J., Wheeler, E., Light, T., Skillings, A., Scharf, M. J., Cropley, T. G., . . . Bernhard, J. D. (1998). Influence of a mindfulness meditation-based stress reduction intervention on rates of skin clearing in patients with moderate to severe psoriasis undergoing phototherapy (UVB) and photochemotherapy (PUVA). *Psychosomatic Medicine, 60*(5), 625-632.

King, M., & Hunt, R. (1967). Dimensions of religiosity in "measuring the religious variable." *Journal for the Scientific Study of Religion, 6*, 173-190.

Koenig, H. G., & Cohen, H. J. (2002). The link between religion and health: Psychoneuroimmunology and the faith factor. New York, NY: Oxford University Press.

Koenig, H. G., George, L. K., & Titus, P. (2004). Religion, spirituality, and health in medically ill hospitalized older patients. *Journal of the American Geriatrics Society, 52*(4), 554-562.

Koenig, H. G., & Larson, D. B. (2001). Religion and mental health: Evidence for an association. *International Review of Psychiatry, 13*, 67-78.

Koenig, H., Parkerson, G. R., Jr., & Meador, K. G. (1997). Religion index for psychiatric research. *American Journal of Psychiatry, 154*, 885-886.

Kosmin, B. A., & Lachman, S. P. (1993). *One nation under God: Religion in contemporary American society.* New York, NY: Harmony Books.

Krause, N. (1998). Stressors in highly valued roles, religious coping, and mortality. *Psychology and Aging, 13*, 242-255.

Krause, N., Chatters, L. M., Meltzer, T., & Morgan, D. L. (2000). Negative interaction in the church: Insights from focus groups with older adults. *Review of Religious Research, 41*, 510-533.

Krause, N., Ellison, C. G., & Wulff, K. M. (1999). Church-based emotional support, negative interaction, and psychological well-being: Findings from a national sample of Presbyterians. *Journal for the Scientific Study of Religion, 37*, 725-741.

Kutner, N. G., Bliwise, D. L., & Zhang, R. (2004). Linking race and well-being within a biopsychosocial framework: Variation in subjective sleep quality in two racially diverse older adult samples. *Journal of Health and Social Behavior, 45*, 99-113.

Larson, D. B., Swyers, J. P., & McCullough, M. E. (1997). *Scientific research on spirituality and health: A consensus report.* Rockville, MD: National Institute for Healthcare Research.

Lee, B. Y., & Newberg, A. B. (2005). Religion and health: A review and critical analysis. *Zygon, 40*(2), 443-468.

Levin, J. (Ed.). (1994). *Religion in aging and health: Theoretical foundations and methodological frontiers.* Thousand Oaks, CA: Sage.

Livingston, I. L., Levine, D. M., & Moore, R. D. (1991). Social integration and Black intraracial variation in blood pressure. *Ethnicity and Disease, 1*, 135-149.

Lo, B., Quill, T., & Tulsky, T. (1999). For the ACP-ASIM End-of-Life Care Consensus Panel. Discussing palliative care with patients. *Annals of Internal Medicine, 130*, 744-749.

MacLean, C. R. K., Walton, K. G., Wenneberg, S. R., Levitsky, D. K., Mandarino, J. P., Waziri, R., . . . Schneider, R. H. (1997). Effects of the transcendental meditation program on adaptive mechanisms: Changes in hormone levels and responses to stress after 4 months of practice. *Psychoneuroendocrinology, 22*(4), 277-295.

Maltby, J., & Day, L. (2003). Religious orientation, religious coping and appraisals of stress: Assessing primary appraisal factors in the relationship between religiosity and psychological well-being. *Personality and Individual Differences, 34*(7), 1209-1224.

Maltby, J., Lewis, C. A., & Day, L. (1999). Religious orientation and psychological well-being: The role of the frequency of personal prayer. *British Journal of Health Psychology, 4*, 363-378.

Mandle, C. L., Domar, A. D., Harrington, D. P., Leserman, J., Bozadjian, E. M., Friedman, R., & Benson, H. (1990). Relaxation response in femoral angiography. *Radiology, 174*(3), 737-739.

Marcer, D. (1986). *Biofeedback and related therapies in clinical practice.* Rockville, MD: Aspen.

Mills, P. J. (2002). Spirituality, religiousness and health: From research to clinical practice. *Annals of Behavioural Medicine, 24*(1), 1-2.

Mirowsky, J., & Ross, C. E. (1992). Age and depression. *Journal of Health and Social Behavior, 33,* 187-205.

Mookherjee, H. N. (1997). Marital status, gender, and perception of well-being. *Journal of Social Psychology, 137,* 95-105.

Pargament, K. I. (1997). *The psychology of religion and coping: Theory, research, practice.* New York, NY: Guilford.

Patel, C., & North, W. R. (1975, July 19). Randomised controlled trial of yoga and bio-feedback in the management of hypertension. *The Lancet, 2,* 93-95.

Patel, C., Marmot, M. G., Terry, D. J., Carruthers, M., Hunt, B., & Patel, M. (1985). Trial of relaxation in reducing coronary risk: Four year follow up. *British Medical Journal, 290,* 1103–1106.

Piccinelli, M., & Wilkinson, B. (2000). Gender differences in depression: Critical review. *British Journal of Psychiatry, 177,* 486-492.

Pollack, A. A., Case, D. B., Weber, M. A., & Laragh, J. H. (1977). Limitations of transcendental meditation in treatment of essential hypertension. *The Lancet, 1*(8002), 71-73.

Ross, C. E., & Van Willigen, M. (1997). Education and the subjective quality of life. *Journal of Health and Social Behavior, 38,* 275-297.

Rozin, P. (2001). Social psychology and science: Some lessons from Solomon Asch. *Personality and Social Psychology Review, 5,* 2–14.

Schmidt, T., Wijga, A., Von Zur Muhlen, A., Brabant, G., & Wagner, T. O. F. (1997). Changes in cardiovascular risk factors and hormones during a comprehensive residential three month kriya yoga training and vegetarian nutrition. *Acta Physiologica Scandinavica: Supplementum, 161,* 158-162.

Schneider, R. H., Nidich, S. I., Salerno, J. W., Sharma, H. M., Robinson, C. E., Nidich, R. J., Alexander, C. N. (1998). Lower lipid peroxide levels in practitioners of the Transcendental Meditation program. *Psychosomatic Medicine, 60*(1), 38-41.

Schneider, R. H., Staggers, F., Alexander, C. N., Sheppard, W., Rainforth, M., Kondwani, K., . . . King, C. G. (1995). A randomized controlled trial of stress reduction for hypertension in older African Americans. *Hypertension, 26,* 820-827.

Scotch, N. A. (1963). Sociocultural factors in the epidemiology of Zulu hypertension. *American Journal of Public Health, 8,* 1205-1213.

Seeman, T. E., Dubin, L. F., & Seeman, M. (2003). Religiosity/

spirituality and health: A critical review of the evidence for biological pathways. *American Psychologist, 58*, 53-63.

Sephton, S. E., Koopman, C., Schaal, M., Thoresen, C., & Spiegel, D. (2001). Spiritual expression and immune status in women with metastatic breast cancer: An exploratory study. *The Breast Journal, 7*, 345-353.

Sephton, S. E., Sapolsky, R. M., Kraemer, H. C., & Spiegel, D. (2000). Diurnal cortisol rhythm as a predictor of breast cancer. *Journal of the National Cancer Institute, 92*, 994-1000.

Seybold, K. S. (2007). Physiological mechanisms involved in spirituality/religiosity and health. *Journal of Behavioral Medicine, 30*, 303-309.

Shaw, B., Han, J. Y., Kim, E., Gustafson, D., Hawkins, R., Cleary, J., . . . Lumpkins, C. (2007). Effects of prayer and religious expression within computer support groups on women with breast cancer. *Psycho-Oncology, 16*, 676-687.

Spilka, B., Hood, R. W., Jr., Hunsberger, B., & Gorsuch, R. (2003). *The psychology of religion: An empirical approach*. New York, NY: Guilford Press.

Stark, R. (2001). *One true God: Historical consequences of monotheism*. Princeton, NJ: Princeton University Press.

Steffen, P. R., Hinderliter, A. L., Blumenthal, J. A., & Sherwood, A. (2001). Religious coping, ethnicity, and ambulatory blood pressure. *Psychosomatic Medicine, 63*, 523-530.

Strawbridge, W. J., Shema, S. J., Cohen, R. D., & Kaplan, G. A. (2001). Religious attendance increases survival by improving and maintaining good health behaviors, mental health, and social relationships. *Annals of Behavioral Medicine, 23*(1), 68.

Sudsuang, R., Chentanez, V., & Veluvan, K. (1991). Effect of

Buddhist meditation on serum cortisol and total protein levels, blood pressure, pulse rate, lung volume and reaction time. *Physiology & Behavior, 50*(3), 543-548.

Sundar, S., Agrawal, S. K., Singh, V. P., Bhattacharya, S. K., Udupa, K. N., & Vaish, S. K. (1984). Role of yoga in management of essential hypertension. *Acta Cardiologica, 39*(3), 203-208.

Timio, M., Lippi, G., Venanzi, S., Gentili, S., Quintaliani, G., Verdura, C., . . . Timio, F. (1997). Blood pressure trend and cardiovascular events in nuns in a secluded order: A 30-year follow-up study. *Blood Pressure, 6*, 81-87.

Underwood, L. G., & Teresi, J. A. (2002). The daily spiritual experience scale: Development, theoretical description, reliability, exploratory factor analysis, and preliminary construct validity using health-related data. *Annals of Behavioral Medicine, 24*, 22-33.

Walsh, A. (1998). Religion and hypertension: Testing alternative explanations among immigrants. *Behavioral Medicine, 24*, 122-130.

Walton, K. G., Pugh, N. D., Gelderloos, P., & Macrae, P. (1995). Stress reduction and preventing hypertension: Preliminary support for a psychoneuroendocrine mechanism. *Journal of Alternative and Complementary Medicine, 1*, 263-283.

Werner, O., Wallace, R., Charles, B., Janssen, G., Stryker, T., & Chalmers, R. (1986). Long-term endocrinologic changes in subjects practicing the Transcendental Meditation and TM-Sidhi program. *Psychosomatic Medicine, 48*(1), 59-66.

Woods, T. E., Antoni, M. H., Ironson, G. H., & Kling, D. W. (1999). Religiosity is associated with affective and immune status in symptomatic HIV-infected gay men. *Journal of Psychosomatic Research, 46*, 165-1

ABOUT THE AUTHORS

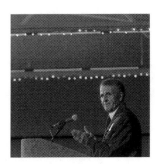

Mohammad R. Torabi, Dean, School of Public Health-Bloomington; Chancellor's Professor, Applied Health Science Department, Indiana University

Kathy L. Finley, MS, Adjunct Faculty, School of Public Health-Bloomington, Applied Health Science Department, Indiana University

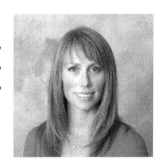

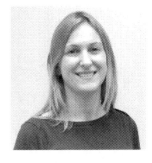

Courtney O. Olcott, M.S., MPH, works as a Prevention Specialist and Research Associate for the Indiana Prevention Resource Center at Indiana University. She is also a doctoral candidate studying Health Behavior in the School of Public Health at Indiana University. Her academic and research interests lie in the area of public mental health and substance abuse prevention.